Rehab

...COLLECTED STORIES AND ESSAYS ON RESOLUTION, RESILIENCY, AND RETURN

BY
SCOTT TINLEY, Ph.D.

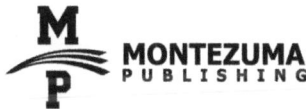

M P
MONTEZUMA PUBLISHING

San Diego, California

Published by Montezuma Publishing - Aztec Shops Ltd.
San Diego State University
San Diego, California 92182-1701
(619) 594-7552
www.montezumapublishing.com

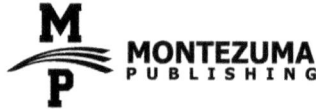

M
P MONTEZUMA
P U B L I S H I N G

ISBN: 978-1-7269-0880-1

Publishing Manager: Lia Dearborn
Production Manager: Steve Murawka
Design & Formatting: Isabella Borquez & Lia Dearborn
Cover Design: Isabella Borquez

Rehab

...COLLECTEDSTORIESAND ESSAYS ON RESOLUTION, RESILIENCY, AND RETURN

BY
SCOTT TINLEY, Ph.D.

... ALSO BY SCOTT TINLEY

Finding the Wheel's Hub:
Tales and Thoughts from the Endurance Athletic Lifestyle

Triathlon:
A Personal History

Racing the Sunset:
An Athlete's Quest for Life After Sport

Things to Be Survived:
Tales of Resolution and Resurrection

Finding Triathlon:
How Endurance Sports Explain the World

In the Wake of Our Past:
A Novel of Historical Fiction

DEDICATION

To my 22; who in her darkest moments became her greater Self

CONTENTS

FOREWORD

I have vivid memories of Scott from the 80s during the peak of his athletic career. A time when I was just a child. My mom would often point to this blonde mustached man on his bike, "there's Scott Tinley riding his bike." Hours later, returning from whatever errand we were on, we'd see that same blonde man, still on his bike. "There's Scott Tinley, still riding his bike." He came to be a man of myth in our community. Running, riding his bike, and ocean swimming with obsessive consistency. Everyone knew it was Scott Tinley when he rode by. He even had a store in the town with his name in lights. But I didn't know him. I knew of him and thought of his abilities as an endurance athlete and as otherworldly and hyper-human. Years later, however, I would come to know him and become his friend; and come to know that the place where all that running and biking and striving came from, was in fact, very human. Especially when he'd falter.

And in fact, his failures, not his achievements, allow him the privilege to write about coming back from that exalted but exhausting place, to be a hero but also a fallen one. To tell the world about his version of rehabilitation. As a M.D. psychiatrist, I can say now that Tinley "earned" the right to talk about rehabilitation not because he was a world champion athlete but he dragged himself up from the parts of life that are quite the contrast to the fame and fortune of athletic supremacy.

Before we met, I left the beach community that we both called home chasing my own adventure. This pursuit culminated with seven months on the Arabian Peninsula, carrying out special operations, and invading a country. When I returned,

I had to re-calibrate myself. I had to give up the familiar and peculiar comforts of my former life—the rhythmic beats of 50 caliber machine guns, the feel of the grip of my rifle, the smells of diesel and gunpowder and sweat. I was without the things that gave me my identity, the sense that I was real and capable. Without it all, I felt somewhat naked and unsure. I had become just an average, regular guy. My own version of rehab.

It was during this time back from my military service that I met Scott. I joined the ranks of the local lifeguard department that he worked for. I can't tell you about the day or the moment we met. In retrospect it seems as though we always knew each other in some way. At that time, I struggled with the sense that no one really appreciated what it was like to be at or in a war one moment and then home the next with a bunch of people who seemed to prefer to be detached from the realities of combat service. I felt minimized, misunderstood, and worlds apart from most people. But Scott seemed to get it. He asked the right questions and reflected ideas and emotions that gave me the impression he knew something about what I was feeling. And he did. Perhaps, more acutely than I can fully appreciate.

The *Tinley* I knew of from my childhood was a man defining himself by his accomplishments and prowess. He became a celebrated figure of human endurance and capability. A bearer of the idea that the human body is capable of far more than anyone appreciates. This became *Tinley*. He battled against himself, and other men, possessed with the idea that their physicality was singularly their own. He had an image of himself—a clear-cut idea of what made him special, different, and meaningful in this world. This, of course, ended. Scott was then forced to see himself, to be himself, and to uncomfortably sit with all he thought was important and what made him real.

I am now an M.D. psychiatrist. A path that was filled with many transitions, recalibrations, and rehabilitations of myself. That path has also put me in a position to be with people during the most challenging moments of their lives. People that are faced with pain so great, that a "leap from the window of the burning building" would bring relief. So many of these people are facing moments that have left them questioning who they are and what they are worth. They have lost themselves. But it is in this time that growth can occur. It is when we have lost who we believed we were that we can finally search and find the essence that makes us who we are. As Henry Thoreau said, "Not until we are lost, do we begin to find ourselves". Some of the most peaceful, self-aware people I know are people who have been to the depths of addiction and reformed themselves from the ashes of despair.

Scott's writing has seemed to always point at this conundrum that we all face in one way or another. To rehabilitate is to "again make fit." At some point in our lives, we must all go through some transition, some change that requires a refitting of our conceptions of self.

Scott's words illustrate all the different forms that *rehab* can take. His collection of writings is a crystalline view of the human struggle against the forces that perpetually try to break us and reform us. Scott's own Hero's Journey has given him the insights to see the world around him through a special lens. He brings humanity and meaning to the struggles and joys of life that others might discount. His gift to the world is his ability to observe the arc of life and recount it with insight, wit, and lasting impression.

—*Nathaniel R. Brown, MD.*

INTRODUCTION

"… he dares to live
Who stops being a bird, yet beats his wings
Against the immense immeasurable emptiness of things."

—T. Roethke, *The Dying Man*

I knew I had slithered into dormancy when my self-winding watch stopped. Days and weeks of lying in stasis, tubes and wires stemming from my body like a science experiment gone horribly wrong had ceased my Timex from ticking. When one of my saintly nurses in the ICU asked me what I would miss the most over the next eight weeks of rehabilitation I told her water; the daily immersion for swimming, surfing … soaking.

"Oh, you mean like that species of shark that needs to swim while sleeping? Don't they need to move oxygenated water through their gills? Just to stay alive?"

"Exactly," I said, asking for another Percocet. "And," riffing on Steinbeck, "good things love water."

The post open-heart surgery (aortic valve replacement) journey had a strange and not-exactly-unwelcomed effect. The sky outside my hospital window seemed bluer, my family gathered as members of a well-trained army unit. Friends who stopped by bearing food and books and secret booze appeared as saviors from across the sea. Nine different meds, five docs, seven nurses, a thousand thoughts on what lie ahead. This is rehab, I concluded; this is a time in your life when you rise from some infantile, pain-racked, helpless blob and ascend to a fully functioning, cognizant, and contributing member of society. In rehab, you get better. Most of the time.

I have tried to hold onto the feelings experienced while I slowly recaptured my humanity. The good, the bad, the ridiculously ugly. I do not want to forget waking up in the ICU, a moment too early, with a tube down my throat. I couldn't breathe; I couldn't speak; only gestures with my barely conscious hands to take that piece of shit out of me. In the future, when I guard the beaches or lecture on drowning, I will remember what it feels like to drown in plain sight. To fight, sometimes helplessly, for your life. I won't forget the nine-out-of-ten pain that was filed off by narcotics and human touch. I won't forget the moments of lucidity, staring at the bright white ceiling thinking it could only get better from here. I won't forget the constant smell of Lysol or the natural born nurses whose ability to heal was forged in tribal history.

When my wife picked me up from the hospital after a week of interment, I sat in the back seat, rolled down the window and put my nose into the wind. No dog could've been happier. Going home meant the first stage in a long and tedious process of rehabilitation and return. Going home meant I wouldn't be living in the beleaguered margins wondering whether my maladies would magically go away or drop me dead on a crowded street, people stepping around the body, asking if I was drunk or homeless. Home meant I could choose the role I wanted to play in this film. Home meant distinguishing the map from the territory.

Home meant health.

═══

In many ways, the concept of "rehab" gets a bad rap. Cloaked in a background of deviance, drugs, alcohol, and general poor choices, the notion of rehabilitation has long been connected to fixing something caused by the victim. Hey, you made your bed. That seems unfair given (most of) the human condition is always and already striving to seek, find, and return to a higher degree of health than the day before. Going into rehab, whether brick and mortar residency, a return from injury and illness, or seeking positive changes to life's myriad choices, rehab might be better looked upon as an action of restoring something that has been damaged to its former (and better) condition.

I didn't think there was anything wrong with my heart. Essentially asymptomatic, I could chalk up the occasional atrial fibrillation to my years as an endurance athlete. I could explain the oh-so-slight decline in cardiac output as age. I was, as the poet said, "Gracefully surrendering the things of youth." I was not unhappy. But as one test led to another and I went down the rabbit hole of results, it became obvious I needed new parts. Refusing to blame it on my athletic choices, my parent's genetic gifts or the fates, I opted to strive for improvement … even before the surgeons sawed my sternum down the middle. Cut me doc, I have an appointment at the cardiac rehab unit four weeks from now. As Admiral Farragut ordered during the battle of Ft. Morgan, "Damn the torpedoes. Full steam ahead."

Isn't it funny how we strive to get better even as we get worse? How we subconsciously know that rehabilitation and all its challenges in our future lie in wait like a benevolent panther in the bush? But getting split stem-to-stern wasn't funny and as the inevitable surgery lie ahead, I sought reasons. As we face the pain related to a journey back to health, we seek reason. Why me? Did I pick my parents wrong? Nope. Was my diet rich in saturated fats? Hardly. Had I ever smoked? Are you kidding me? What about your years as a professional endurance athlete? Oh, maybe there was a connection.

From 1982 to 1999, my primary profession was listed on the tax return as "professional athlete" which meant I got paid to swim, bike, and run. Good work, if you can get it. The reality was, however, it was hard. An average week included 350 miles of cycling, 75 miles of running, 30,000 yards of swimming, and all the ancillary efforts such as strength training, stretching, and medical care. Not much time to sneak in those rehabilitative afternoon naps. So, nearly 100 victories, and two world championships later, I was bone tired. And my heart, as a primary and necessary muscle, had been ridden hard and put up wet. 25 years later, some of the parts wore out. Oops. Welcome to cardiac rehab.

——

One of the beautiful curses of the rehabilitation process is that no two returns to normalcy are ever the same. Playbooks may exist ranging from 12-Step to tough love to incarceration, each with its own set of rules and rubrics. But in our often deeply personal struggles to shake hands across the Great Divide that is sustainable health and everything else, we can wonder about this meandering irony. Some folks go into the rehab journey armed with bunkers of commitment and resources. Others deny the issue. More than a few will dabble a toe or two. And for some, like Jim MacLaren, rehab isn't a thing to go through but a part of their post-accident identity.

In the summer of 1985, the new Yale-minted grad was hit by a New York City bus and pronounced DOA. "After my heart started beating again," Jim recalled, "I wondered why they had chalked the outline of my body." MacLaren lost a leg in that accident but rehabilitated his body and spirit back into running a 3:16 marathon. Tragically, eight years later while competing in a triathlon, Jim was struck by another vehicle and rendered a mid-level quadriplegic. Confined to a wheelchair for the rest of his short life (he died in on August 31st, 2010), MacLaren was in constant motion searching for pain relief, searching for acceptance if not love, and trying to make sense of the skull-and-crossbones existence he'd been given. For twenty-five of his forty-seven years, Jim MacLaren was in rehab.

The other bad wrap that rehab gets is how most people reduce it to chemical or behavior-centricity. The devil twins of drugs and alcohol. Did we forget that life messes with the mighty and the weak and the middle-man as they all struggle to deal with a failed relationship, a broken link in their mental processes, a loss of spiritual belief, a lost job, a lost child, a loss of belief in anything good? To rehabilitate oneself is to restore that which is broken or damaged or missing or somehow completely fucked up by injury, illness, addiction, war, loss, gain, too much, too little, excitement, boredom, money, poverty, family, friends and all the beautiful vagaries that are part of the human existence.

Rehab ain't just going on the wagon. Substance abuse is a disease that needs to be treated as such, no differently than depression, suicidal tendencies, anxiety, domestic violence, and obesity. Equal opportunity rehabilitation.

Still, more often than not when people think about rehab, addiction comes to mind. Which suggests these are fallible and weak characters who can't seem to follow Nancy Reagan's advice and just say no. And these unending "choices" made by those who *mostly* in their cogent minds, seek and find a vehicle to alter the way they feel with legal and illegal substances, get tossed into the category of deviance. *They need to go into rehab*, we argue, because they are breaking the law. I am a university-level teacher, a grandfather, a tax-paying property owner, and a respected member of my community who volunteers for various causes. I use caffeine, statins, acetaminophen, alcohol, herbs, Ibuprofen, bees wax, sugar, potassium, naproxen, and copious amounts of garlic daily to improve my mood and seek better health. I could hardly be labeled a drug user. If I eliminated any or all the above elements, would I need to enter a rehab facility? Would I face jail time? Public social stoning by my peers?

======

With those ideas in mind, and as I was negotiating my return from open heart surgery, I set about writing, curating, and collecting new, old, and re-written essays and stories that addressed rehabilitation from perhaps a fresh and organic perspective. I wanted to connect rehab with restoration, resiliency with reformation, and a possible return with some new-found feelings about people's lives as they navigated death and divorce, helplessness, hope, and health. I wanted to use these stories and essays as vehicles to help explain things like the randomness of illness and injury, the slippery timelines, pain management, the way that we are re-situated in a different state when we face the beautifully cold and harsh realities. I wanted to explore rehabilitation as if it was the game and we were a big game hunter.

Rehab can range from cancerous, soul-sucking bone pain lit by a single, swaying, sixty-watt bulb in your tenement basement to a month-long stay in a posh, hillside, mocktail-serving Malibu "facility," that caters to the victims of such first-world maladies as sex addiction and gambling concerns. The similarities might surprise you; carryovers reminding them that rain falls on the just and the unjust.

Perhaps rehabilitation is the most egalitarian part of human suffering.

The concept of rehabilitation—from beating the odds, from beating drugs and disease and death and all the shit that life throws at us—can be a grand opportunity or our final undoing. There is much involved in this most human of endeavors.

—S.T.

SECTION 1:

THE REHAB FROM EVENTS THAT WENT WRONG

Introduction

On the morning of June 3rd, 2024, I was opening the main lifeguard tower in my hometown of Del Mar, California. That was my shift. It was around 7:45AM and a small group of regular swimmers were starting to show up for their weekly ocean swim. The weather was typical June Gloom, overcast, with south winds steady at 6-8 knots. The surf was 2-4 feet, and the ocean was not very inviting. One of the swimmers looked disgusted by the conditions and shook his head. Setting up the requisite flags and cones on the beach, I made small talk with the swimmer.

"Hey, there aren't many surfers to get in your way, the water is a balmy 65* and the currents are mild. Looks like a decent day to swim with your pals. What could go wrong?"

Just under an hour later, one of the swimmers, Caleb Adams, 46-year-old, was bitten several times by what was later identified as a 12-foot white shark. He survived the ordeal and has returned to ocean swimming. How Adams was able to rehab physically, mentally, and emotionally must still be an unfolding negotiation within his mind and his body.

As we rehab the things that challenge us, we ask not just, "What could go wrong?" But more importantly, "Why did that happen to me?"

Losing our youth is unavoidable. But what happens when the unexpected reaches out and grabs us, pulls us under and kills just a part of us? We're still breathing but maybe we're confined to a wheelchair or incarcerated, or a part of our heart has left us along with our favorite dog. What happens when the things and the people and the places and everything we believe in goes away? The likelihood seems as impossible as two commercial jet liners flying into New York skyscrapers.

How do we return from a dead-end street that has no place to turn around? In this section we get to climb inside the head and the heart of those who did and those who didn't turn around without hitting the curb. And those who are still trying.

Prescript: *On a national scale, I can think of no single post-modern event that has catalyzed the need for emotional, physical, and spiritual rehab than the events of 9/11/2001. It changed America in ways the average person may not have any concept of, altering our way of life more than anything except WWII and COVID. Decades later we still wrestle with the question, "Is the U.S.A. a better country than before 9/11?" It appears that the great majority have mostly healed from this horrific day. Still, there are others in perpetual rehab, who can never and should never forget. And too many that will never find peace. Question of rehab are extended during a global crisis such as 9/11. Were there root problems that America missed? Signs of the impending disaster? Does blame and retribution make us heal better? Quicker? More fully? Was culpability ever fully exhumed? Did you hate Arabs for a while? And here we are, several decades hence trying to figure out where such hatred and malevolence were born. In perhaps one of the most rehabilitative moments in this century, when Osama Bin Laden's dead body was on a U.S. naval ship returning from operations in the Middle East, his body was thrown over the side. There were some who wanted to see the dead murderer paraded through the streets of NYC while thousands could claim victory over Al Qaeda. President Obama, arguing for calm if not national security, said, "We don't need to spike the football."*

Start with 343

> *"When ignorance erodes any trace of memory it becomes possible to declare that history demands the lie be made sacred and indisputable. Yet history seems to be a relentless pursuer."*
>
> —Steven Schmidt, 9/8/21

> *"There's an old poster out west. It says, 'wanted dead or alive' ... I want justice."*
>
> —President George W. Bush, 9/20/2001

343 NYC firefighters lost their lives on that horrific day on September 11th of 2001. Over 350 additional have died since due to related injuries and illnesses.

For a period, the notion of what constitutes a "hero" had changed in America. Tiger Woods and the Kardashians were replaced by paramedics and firefighters and nurses and cops and lifeguards. Everyday people are going about their daily lives, saving others who might lose theirs.

It was a Phoenix moment for our country. We would never forget. We'd learn from our mistakes. To serve the memory of those who had died at the hands of ignorance, evil and misanthropy ... America would be better.

And then we followed the advice of Cheney, Bush, and Rumsfeld. We invaded Iraq looking for weapons of mass destruction. We initiated "enhanced interrogation" at Guantanamo. We stayed in Afghanistan for another 20-plus years, the result being America now has 14 times the number of terrorist group enemies than we had in 2001. Had America failed to heed the advice of Rev. Nathan Baxter as he addressed those at the memorial service for 9-11 victims at Washington's National Cathedral on September 16, 2001, quoting Congresswoman Barbara Lee, "Let us not become the evil we deplore in the search for justice."

Yes, revenge matters because there are humans amongst us who fail to comprehend rules of law, who have degraded our worlds with their ignorance and self-serving ideology. But a more rational response might be "How better to respond to conflict than with compassion?" Then again, I only lost a few peripheral friends in the attack. Had I lost a loved one, I might've suggested nuclear response or as one military leader said, "Let's bomb the region into the Stone Age." The question still begs, if Osama Bin Laden were alive today, would he feel that he accomplished his mission not just with bombs and planes but with the concepts of Gitmo and drone strikes and failure of adherence to the Geneva Convention and habeas corpus and frontier justice response? Undocumented workers with a tattoo and an Oakland Raiders hat shipped to prisons in El Salvador.

One of the problems is that radicalized terrorists don't fear death the way most thoughtful Westerners do. Perhaps an observable generation interred in horrible places like Guantanamo Bay and darker dungeons around the world have been a deferment to post 9/11 attacks. What are the human costs to find out though?

If evil and revenge are a concept, then isn't democracy and education and rationality just as conceptual?

The attacks of 9/11, the first to fully occur on American soil in our country's history, were the single most catastrophic since the Civil War. But have we fully realized the 20-plus-year ripples of those heavy rocks?

God and Allah. Heaven and hell. The Yankees and the Red Sox. Capitalism and socialism. Going straight home after work or stopping at the pub for a round. Red hats vs. blue hats.

When I think about the 343 NYC firefighters, these eclectic polarities come to mind as we navigate our own negotiations between our beliefs and our responses. The 343 were beyond modern herodom because post-modern media heroes, like 9/11 itself, have become a commodified item, bought and sold on the market. The firefighters of the NYFD didn't have time to over-think and were trained to act calmly and without judgment.

Three decades as a beach lifeguard have allowed me enough tenure to show unadulterated respect for the fallen. And wonder at how the NYFD has kept focus on bravery, on duty, on the men and women who gave their lives in service of those in need. How the people of NYC aren't citing similarities or differences between the Quran and the Old Testament but instead, singing sustainable praise for the pure humanity shown by its first responders.

That horror cannot be unlived. But what we've done or can still do with 9/11 may guide us in perpetuity. If you want to understand what Al-Qaeda did or did not do to America, start with the 343.

Prescript: First published in Finding Triathlon (Hatherleigh Press, 2015), I tried to make sense of growing older as an athlete, of losing speed, and flexibility, power, and performance. I never wanted to end up a Glory Days guy, regaling stories at the pub like Stallone in Rocky 5. With some fortune, I had a handful of older mentors who early schooled me in what to keep and what to discard. Leaving a long tenure as a professional athlete, I was wrestling with issues of identity and direction. I distinctly remember meeting a retired NFL player who had studied athlete transition. One of the first things he said to me after we shook hands and ordered coffee was, "Scott, the sooner you realize the best part of your life is over, the sooner you can move on to having a pretty good second half." It seemed harsh but in retrospect, it was brilliantly poignant and offered a perspective beyond what my confused mind would allow. As the weeks, months, and years unfolded and I found new ways of being in the world beyond sport, I came to appreciate how we too often equate happiness with occupational success, a good life with a good body. The ideas below reflect my attempt to make sense of the pathetic fallacy that only the young, strong, and beautiful can truly be happy.

Aging Up

My neighbor John can't run anymore. The soft tissue around his knees isn't torn, tattered, ripped or scarred. It's just gone; like some magician from his youth had waved a handkerchief over his leg and *shazam*—thirty-thousand miles later, the head of the tibia is staring at the lower part of the femur like two grumpy old neighbors. The soft tissue and the ivy-laden fence gone, they must redefine their relationship.

The cool part about John is that he's okay with it.

"This knee has supported me for much longer than I would've expected," he spoke, as if giving a eulogy for a fallen soldier. "He's contributed to the cause, done his time and now I'll let him rest."

I almost wanted to take my hat off and sing Amazing Grace.

The relationship that some athletes have with their body is like that of a jilted love: you only really understand it when you feel the bone-level pain of unexpected loss. It's justifiable, of course. The musculoskeletal and cardiovascular systems that propel us—as 250-pound linebackers, forward into human carnage; as seven-foot forwards, upward into rarefied air; and as endurance athletes, across barren lava fields—is the vehicle that provides us with not only our recreation but our identity. The embodied athlete finds validity as a human being with a particular purpose. For the athlete, arms and legs aren't body parts; they're an extension of our psyche and our soul.

And so, it is when appendages and central parts fail the athlete, we are rarely unaffected. Career-ending surgeries can bring depression and necessary adjustment of self-identity. Minor strains and sprains cause irritability and frustration. My neighbor's level of appreciation and acceptance is an anomaly. The insightful and pragmatic will realize that the athlete's relationship with their body is as fluid and dynamic as the body itself, much more so than the sedentary individual. How we think about our bodies is affected by intrinsic and extrinsic factors, self-images from within and mediated images from the outside.

Athletes' bodies have become part of the economic and cultural landscape. It's not only about skill and performance anymore. It's about just looking good while we do it. Athlete's bodies are objectified, aestheticized, and commodified. In other words, they are separated from the human as a living being, looked upon as art and beauty and then sold in every form from the masculinized Gladiator to a sexualized pin-up doll. If you aren't talented enough to win but you have the goods elsewhere, you can still become a talking-head commentator or star in a centerfold spread.

The body has many roles to play, and society is often the curtained puppeteer holding the strings. But we all have a little Pinocchio in us—that innate need to go it alone. We are tossed into the fray of decisions. What do we think of our bodies? Are they simply a carrier for our minds and souls? Are they meant to carry us across oceans and continents and finish lines and the bathroom floors? Are they meant to attract a sexual partner and if the gods are smiling, procreate the species? Or some unanswerable amalgamation of the above?

Elite athletes have a reputation for narcissism, for an overt focus on how they appear while they perform. Any number of participants will justify this with comments like, "I worked hard to look this good, to go this fast. I'll flaunt it as much as I want." To be sure, there is nothing wrong with showing outward pride in the results of inward hard work. It's natural. What's problematic is when our feelings toward our bodies and what we can or cannot do with them become manipulated by those who may not have our own best interests at heart. Still, endurance sport athletes have shown a level of independence in thought and action. There is little difference between a teenager with a purple Mohawk and the first Ironman competitors. Somebody said it couldn't or shouldn't be done. And so, they went and did it.

At what cost though? Serious triathletes have often traded health for fitness, only learning the difference when tragedy comes knocking as a stress fracture or chronic fatigue. Or worse.

There are people like Rudy Garcia-Tolsen, whose story is well-known, and Dr. Beck Wethers of the infamous 1996 Mt. Everest tragedy when five climbers died in a sudden storm. The Dallas physician, who lost all or parts of several fingers, toes and facial parts, reportedly told an interviewer who'd inquired about the multiple challenges he faced without digits and dexterity, "It's only body parts."

Indeed. But those parts are hard to come by, even with reconstructive surgery. Wethers and Garcia-Tolsen, who opted to have his deformed legs removed as a child so that he could "Be more like the other kids," certainly took the high road. But the conversation on surgeries necessarily needs to be separated by notions of need. I admire females that opt for breast reduction when it serves their athletic lifestyle or any other desire for self-improvement. Still, so many females must feel challenged when set up against elective surgery that alters such socially-inscribed maladies as size 32 B breasts and replaces them with a set of media-fueled, desirable 36 D twins; one wonders just how any of us might go about this relationship with our bodies as society influences our desire for a shape that is attractive to a mate. And sometimes we might ask why the public discussion on elective surgery rarely includes males who choose penis, pectoralis or calf muscle augmentation. Why no discussion on a male Baywatch character for his skinny legs and receding hair line? But if the elective option, at any level for any reason, rekindles lost feelings of self-esteem, and results in better lives, how can we not celebrate what modern medicine can do? There are no right or wrong answers, only personal choices.

I hope that when my joints grind away like chalkboard fingernails and my face looks like the dashboard of a '62 Buick left out in the Arizona sun, and my kids have to help me onto my three wheeled bicycle, I will be able to say that she gave me a good ride.

Other days, I remember when it didn't. When it was busted.

Growing Older, Not Up

The body in sport is a vehicle for learning how we are in the world, something to be enjoyed, cherished, and well-considered. I've noted that as endurance athletes we often abuse it, but our bodies reward us all the same. The human body doesn't suck.

Until it grows old.

Aging up in sport is like in-laws: they come in all shapes and sizes and some you can stand to have around longer than others. With the injuries of age, for example, I don't know if the little teasers like a strained this and sprained that, a wrinkle here and sunspot there, all wrought through our obsession for fitness and submission to time are any better than the serious injuries that force us to put our feet up and actually read a book or talk with friends without worrying that we might be late for swim practice. But they cause us concern and remind us of the humanness of the human body.

We do our best to push those days beyond the horizon because the body really is an amazing thing. As fragile and resilient and wondrous as it is, it ain't perfect. Like ugly dogs and poorly written songs, it needs love. But we don't want to be servants to them either. The toothpaste commercials remind us of that youthful exuberance, well-oiled joints, and blinding smiles are an omnipotent refraction of health. Still, left to bake under that desert sun, the dry meatless skull holding those teeth in place, they'll bleach to the same shade. And we'll be long gone, your neighbor and you swapping old training stories and fish tales.

It would be nice to know how to get old though. Without injuries.

Now, you can certainly read the books and listen to the sod-busting silverbacks as they weave stories, and swap lies down at the corner shop. But to truly know how to be an older jock with an injury you have to be, well ... older.

Fair enough, you might think. But is knowing how to gracefully surrender the things of youth a white flag wave of submission or a white light of wisdom?

It seems that we are engaged in a temporal/cultural arms race of sorts. As society continues to embrace all things young, a correlative supply of youth-making activities, diets, devices, and drugs are meeting market demands. Or at least they allow us to look good enough in dim light and heavy rouge to convince a buyer. Currently we are at a push, with mutual détente the goal-old enough to borrow money, vote and drink but without the crow's feet, furrowed brow, and forced compromise. And while the male and female boomers or various age groups cling with desperation to the faux myth of twenty-something, pouring themselves into tight jeans, red Ferraris, Botox, and a Tindered relationship, the Great Hands of Time sweep them further into this vicarious flirt with their past.

Less than two hundred years ago, my age (late fifty-something, sort of) would be considered a full life by most standards. Age has become a relative thing, however. And even though Time still moves at the same speed (give or take a few very minor adjustments) we move faster, racing from one time-saving meeting to another time-efficient, health-promoting workout; all the while trying to fend off the recasting of memory, that sure-fire road to the bane of rose-tinted nostalgia. It is better that we save it all for the armchair years when we can re-wind the tape and tweak the results to our favor.

Everybody loves old people. We just don't want to be one.

How self-deceiving that we should force-tune our minds to a hip-hop score when classic rock or even Muzak is what our advancing cells crave. All we've done is create our own stereotypes, allow Madison Ave. to be the architect of our desires and, quite likely, increase our aging in the process. It's the tortoise and the hare with a Sisyphean sub-plot.

Yet not everyone lives with tin foil on their windows. Growing older as an athlete places you in the company of others who know how to walk that high wire of aging-up, how to live in a societal DMZ on a raft between the phalanxes of illusory youth and the rocky shores of unnecessary debilitation; a place that has to be earned, appreciated, and accepted. With a bit of wind, it can be a lovely sail.

You've met them. They know the constellation of possibilities that come with titles like Grand Master and Kahuna. They don't freak out when a notice from the AARP arrives in the mail. They celebrate birthdays replete with enough candles to set off the smoke alarm. They reserve silicone for caulking the bathtub. They train less but smarter, refusing to consider their commitment to athleticism as one might be obligated to stations of the cross or a serial monogamous relationship with one route, one sport, one way to keep the blood flowing. Old, smart jocks worship Jimmy Buffet and grow older, not up. They are their own tribe of weathered refugees, happy to be in motion because their arterial flow is fueled not by the media or by golden-calf, ill-motivated, five-hour bike rides. Only by the knowledge that they could do it and still be at their desks by noon, fresh and ready to design better widgets.

It's hard to meld the past with the future, to exist in the moment with one foot in Gen-X and the other in gentrification. But sport is a kind of friction-free lubrication, a bridge that not so much spans time as it elongates the moments between then and now. Through sport we can play hopscotch on the sidewalk and shun the dystopia of SUV-consciousness. Through sport we can wear those tight jeans because larger ones fall and anything medium has a vanilla taste. Through sport we can move laterally, dancing between worlds, generations, leaping like spawning salmon or bottom-lying, ageless catfish. Through sport we can move through time with grace instead of youthful rage or desolate, perimenopausal cynicism.

I suppose that learning how to know how a life-long process is. In the beginning you succeed on instinct. Closer to the end you win because you just don't give a damn. Ever wonder why kids and grandparents never tuck their shirts into their pants while the mid-term, over-achievers wear flip-top cell phones on leather belts that match their shoes? I'd like to think that I'm smarter than my training log, heart rate monitor and rear-view mirror. I know that appearing objects are potentially larger than what I see or measure. And I pray that if I keep in shape with training by feel, ambition, and some hopeful interpretation of dreams, I will be able to cast off the shackles of immaturity and arrive time and again at the place that I've come to know as the beginning.

Prescript: David Bailey was the first physically challenged friend I had that simultaneously made me both calm, thrilled, and nervous to be around. I wasn't sure why. Perhaps it was because his injury had hit close to home. (I'd fractured part of my vertebrae in a mountain bike crash and walked away). Or the way he had, at first, refused to believe he wouldn't walk again. I had initially encountered Bailey in the mid-80s when he was a national motocross champion and was dabbling a toe in the world of triathlons as a format to gain physical fitness for his grueling sport. David was good looking, talented, intelligent, and was earning a high six-figure income. He was recently married to a beautiful woman, and was on top of the offroad motorcycle racing world. And then he crashed and burned during practice for a non-consequential race in January of 1987. Over the years we stayed in touch, and I'd watch his metamorphosis with quiet awe. His battles with disbelief and depression, bed sores, finding a new career, staying married, winning the Ironman World Championship in the wheelchair division, raising a family ... all suggest what kind of man, if not person, Bailey was. David was struggling with the same things that most of us do as we move through life's periods.

But he was doing it from a wheelchair.

Over the years I've tried to wrap my head around how difficult that transition must've been. But I can't. The closest I came was 90 days after my fractured C6 vertebrae had healed. My orthopedic surgeon pulled me aside and said, "well, you can do anything you want now. No limitations." I think I was looking for something more worldly from him, a "good luck" and "Godspeed" kind of thing. So, I prompted him with well, I know I'm lucky and then he stopped, put his hand on my shoulder, turned toward the door slowly and said, "Mr. Tinley, every day I see people of all ages who get wheeled into the OR on gurneys. Many of them will never have full use of their extremities again. And their method of injury was less traumatic than yours. What you do with the rest of your able-bodied life is up to you. Have a nice day."

It took me a long time to ask David to revisit his journey. I supposed it's kind of like asking someone about the details of a car crash or a messy divorce or losing a child. Some things are just left buried. But I sensed he might be willing to go there for this project. When he sent me this tome with a small apology for its length and tardiness and something like, "It was cathartic," I knew I was in for a ride. His mentor, fellow wheelchair racer Jim Knaub, had recently passed away and I think the notion of mortality had crept in. Perhaps Bailey was reminded of the much lower life expectancy of the physically challenged. Perhaps he was finally ready to walk us through his rehab.

Here I Am: David Bailey's Most Unlikely Journey

ST: *What was your first reaction when you were told that you wouldn't walk again?*

This Dr. Wilmot came into my hospital room, seemingly frustrated because nurses or whoever indicated that I was still wanting to know when I could get up and start doing something to get better. He was there to say, what's this I hear? I then re-asked, "When can I start making some progress? How long? What's next?" His reply, best I can remember was, "You have damaged your spinal cord, and you will never walk again … so I suggest you understand that and start listening to the PT's and learn how to take care of yourself in this condition so we can release you to go home and be able to function." My reaction? Disbelief. I wasn't mad, sad, just in shock. It was terrible news, but not totally because I didn't consider it as final. He doesn't know "me." I'm not some guy who got stabbed in a gang war, or some drunk driver who wrecked his car. I'm a professional athlete who has overcome the standard news of; you'll be in a cast for four to six weeks. For example, I had my eyes opened to a broken fibula as something I could still stand on and race with if I could handle the pain. I could race with broken feet or a ruined ankle because of the desire to win. Dr. Wilmots terrible news was in my opinion, *only his* opinion. So, it didn't affect me right away. I only thought I was for sure not going to be okay by the first race, but maybe later in the year to defend my 500cc championship. I figured once out of that hospital I would get different news and things to begin doing to start getting better.

ST: *Did you have any kind of support system (family, friends, outside interests) that enabled you through those early dark times?*

Yes, I had a great support system. Gina, my mom who flew from Virginia to Santa Clara, California near San Jose where I was for 3 1/2 months, my dad Gary at times, and locals who learned I was there and showered me with everything from Bibles to cookies, to a smoothie to simply being there and visiting with nothing but positivity. My mechanic, some Honda personnel, good friends from back east made the trip as well and my real dad Terry Martin who drove all the way in an old Ford van from Dana Point. My teammate Johnny O'mara, his girlfriend (Gina's friend), and Drew Lein who started a company called 100%, fan mail that filled a shopping cart daily and even Dave Scott who drove over from Davis in a heavy thunderstorm. Tons of support! However, few of them knew what I was actually facing. Through ignorance, (well-meaning though) I heard things like, "if anyone can beat this it's you! You're a champion. You can do it. Just stay positive." I would just have to dig deeper because this was a bigger and more drastic hurdle, but eventually I'd get over it and have an inspiring comeback story I thought. Those who had an idea (of my condition) were in for a real shock. Or maybe they didn't want to be the ones to break it to me. Plus, who really knows? What Dr. Wilmot knew and perhaps some others was that I was in denial. I believed I could get better, get up and walk and get back out there and ride like the wind.

ST: How did your ventures into "alternative" modes of healing affect your overall rehabilitation?

I eventually left the hospital and Gina drove me down the California coast in my west coast vehicle, a red Toyota pickup, to our townhouse in Simi Valley which was home base on the west coast near the Honda test track (Hondaland) and a couple miles from my teammate O'Mara. In my mind I would start doing treatments again with Dr Martin and his son in Pasadena. Our Honda team trainer, Jeff Spencer had introduced me to alternative methods to treat injuries, and they worked. I credit Jeff for several championships because had I listened to regular doctors I would have been in a cast, crutches, surgeries, etc. and not won a Supercross title or an outdoor national or a Wrangler Grand National Championship. So, in my mind the work would begin, and I would be on the road to recovery! But two things happened, first, as Gina pulled up to our townhouse and the garage door slowly went up, there was my Eclipse carbon bicycle with Roval wheels that I just had built and raced at the Desert Princess Duathlon in Palm Springs, my running shoes, and my practice bike. I lost it! Tears, reality, and a sudden horrible feeling washed over me like a nightmare, except I was awake. It became real. A little bit of doubt crept in. Second, a long and real conversation over the phone with Jeff Spencer.

During that phone conversation, I was telling him all I planned to do as if that was where I needed to place 100% of my thoughts and efforts. Back to Dr. Martin and if that back-and-forth trip from Simi Valley proved to be too much, I'd just buy a diathermy machine and ultrasound and go full blast! Jeff's reply though surprised me. He said, "But what if that doesn't work?" Hmm. Yeah, but I'm going to this and that and Jeff said again, "I know, but … what if that doesn't work?" He must've listened to me for at least an hour convincing myself. And would say again, I know David, but what if all those things and efforts and machines don't work? I'll never forget it. I wasn't mad, I wasn't depressed or rocked, but it got my attention. Jeff was the first person to question it all and suggest, perhaps this might be it - and if so, will I be able to accept that? I heard him, I trusted him, but being in denial and feeling like I owed it to myself, my brand-new wife - who had learned while I was still in the hospital that she was pregnant - my family, team and fans to at least try and I did! I bought those machines and kept my hopes up. Hey, maybe I'll be walking by the time our new baby is. Gotta stay positive I thought, as did many friends and fans. After months of learning how to go to the bathroom and function, none of which I paid attention to in rehab at the hospital because I wasn't going to need that anyway, I finally was up for a cross-country flight back to our real house in Axton, VA. to settle in. My family and awesome group of friends and a couple current racers were all there making our house accessible! A new downstairs add-on with a master bedroom, bathroom and ramps were completed, and Gina and I flew back. I wasn't as devastated as I was when I returned to Simi Valley, I'd already been through those emotions and was more mentally prepared, but there was definitely a funk. I had a friend/chiropractor from Florence, SC, who believed he could help me. He had a trailer full of machines and stayed parked in my driveway and went to work on me daily. Adjustments, acupuncture, and everything you could imagine. I still had hope, but nothing was changing yet. Information did not exist for a T4 and T5 Thoracic SCI and what to do. All that existed was reality and wheelchairs and shower and commode benches and ramps. Every case was different so I pressed on thinking, "I" could give it 100% and break through. If anyone could, I felt qualified because I wasn't going to accept it and give up. Then I learned of the Miami Project headed up by Nick Buoniconti and his son who was a quadriplegic and was developing a new program in Miami with biofeedback and electric stem bikes to keep your legs in shape. It was a group of supposedly the best doctors worldwide sharing information to find a cure. The lead doctor was Dr Barth Green who I met, and he looked at all my x-rays and said, "Well you can see here that your spinal cord isn't cut, just badly bruised." That's what I wanted to hear so we rented a place in Key Biscayne, where our son Sean who was born in Oct,

'87. He was with us, and I stayed there in paradise for several more months giving it 100%! Yet still, there was no change.

ST: Was there an "a ha" moment when you realized that you had to move on with your life, realize your future in a chair, and just get over the guilt or depression that may have been holding you back?

After the Miami project, we returned to Virginia, and I even flew off to Fort Collins Colorado once to a doctor who claimed he had a technique that could make all the difference. It was a massive let down! When I returned from that trip with Gina I was devastated and I could see Gina was fully aware I was trying anything from bullshit marketing, to quacks all selling hope, but it was false. Wham! I got dark. Gina was getting tired of it. I knew it but still I couldn't stop whining and making it no fun for anyone around. I didn't want to live anymore. It got that bad. She decided to go visit her family in Vermont and let them all see our son Sean and give me some time to bitch all by myself and hopefully get it out of my system! Then the most surprising thing was that I rented a movie called *Joe Versus the Volcano*. I was trying to laugh and keep things upbeat. Partway into that movie, Tom Hanks, who was wasting his life and decided to sacrifice himself by jumping into a volcano, ends up floating on some luggage at sea. One night, sunburned, thirsty, hallucinating a little bit, it suddenly dawns on him, and he looks at a humongous moon and says, "Dear God whose name I do not know, thank you for my life! I never realized." At that exact moment, I realized if I knew when it was going to end, what would I be doing with my remaining time? The answer? Stop complaining, start exercising, start doing things myself, get my license and start driving and start doing "something!" So, I did. Weights, pushing my chair a few miles over to my parents' house up a gravel road in the Virginia heat and humidity. I knew how to exercise. That was free. I didn't need a machine or a doctor. I could simply lift weights, stretch, and push my chair. From there my attitude changed. I still kept my hopes up for some cure or medical miracle, but I wasn't only focused on that. I was living again and Gina returned to the man she married, sort of. One night in bed in the dark I said to Gina, "Do you want to move to California and start fresh?" YES!!!! Immediately the next day we (she) began making arrangements for our "stuff" to be trucked to Carlsbad, CA. And we boarded a flight to the 1989 Hawaii Triathlon with our son Sean. When the race/vacation was over we would fly back to San Diego and get our stuff and figure it out.

ST: Were you able to identify certain personal, behavioral traits that provided you with the resiliency or courage or tenacity to go on?

What set me apart from the rest in motocross was (IMO) the desire to find a newer and more effective way. Better preparation, better technique, working harder at it, doing more than the rest. Make it work! But that ability to figure things out and blaze a new trail and not quit, maybe make adjustments, but never quit was also my worst enemy because expected results, but physically I wasn't getting any. I was renting a hotel room at Pea Soup Andersons in Carlsbad and training with extra motivation having just been to Ironman while we looked for a house. I also started a job. I would drive from the house we were renting to Chula Vista and JT Racing USA, the riding gear manufacturer that I wore when I raced. They were the Nike of motocross gear and protection and the owner/founder, and his wife put me to work. If I could still race, what would I want to wear? What colors, what is missing? What would I like to see? As I was doing that and actually making some money again John Gregory, the owner could see I was doing pretty good, but maybe I wasn't quite as adjusted as the fellow Jim Knaub he sponsored who was injured similarly; he was a 3-time winner of the Boston marathon and an actor in shows like Happy Days, Fall Guy, and various commercials, and seemingly not bothered a bit by his disability. So, one day in early 1990 I show up for work and parked in my handicap spot next to a convertible Rambler with two racing chairs sticking up out of the back seat. Now we're talking! Those look good I thought compared the ones I had seen up until then. I met John in his office, and there sits Jim Knaub who I knew nothing about. But he wasn't sitting in his chair, he was sitting in one of John's big leather office chairs and his wheelchair was over to the side. He was strong, handsome, seemed pretty sharp and he took one look at me and the tough love started. I accepted. I didn't mind. Whatever way he made fun of my florescent pink, yellow and pearl white chair I painted to look like Kenny Sousa's bicycle or my Dodge caravan with a lift or any bit of whining on my part, I realized he was right. I realized he knew what he was talking about and could kick my ass in every category so I listened, because for the first time since I crashed in January of 1987, I met somebody who was adjusted, kicking ass and willing to take me under his wing so I absorbed whatever criticism he had and any ideas he had, first of which was a trip to Cabo. It was there that the shower chair, toilet chair, complaining, "I can't" all disappeared into, what I "could" do! Jim knew there was an athlete in there, I just needed to be activated, and a racing wheelchair was step one. Quit worrying about what you can't do and start focusing on what you can do he would say. I needed a push from somebody who did know what a SCI was and had adjusted and was willing to show me. So, I went from pushing my chair a couple miles for exercise, to hauling ass in a racing wheelchair 30 miles a week, racing local 10Ks, marathons, a job, and a new son. We found a house in Vista and in the early 90's ESPN called asking if I would be interested in doing color commentary on TV for outdoor motocross races and I said yes! I didn't even ask what it paid, I just knew I was going to have to figure out by myself how to fly back and forth across the country, get a rental car, stay in a hotel and look presentable on TV and if I said yes, I would HAVE to! I was on a roll and building momentum and had another job. Plus, Gina said, "I'm pregnant again!" We didn't know we could have kids but evidently, we could. Our son Sean was three and we learned he would have a sister. From not wanting to live to stepping out and taking chances, I was living again. Working, racing, designing, being a husband, and a father. Who knows what's next?

ST: How about setbacks? Were there times when you thought you were getting better and then something happened to move you back into anxiety or depression? That "why me?" syndrome? Talk about your interest in sports and dirt bikes and triathlons. Would you say that in some ways, those other interests enabled your rehab?

For years, racing against other people in similar conditions, not one of them was the same. No same injury and injury level and different sensations and pain or lack of it. Some could have kids, some couldn't. Some were on fire with pain that no meds could touch while others didn't have any, but one thing was consistent, pressure sores! I made it a decade without any setbacks. I heard some horror stories, but I always chalked it up to, "Well that's because he did this or that and I don't." I'm an athlete who, by then, had gone back to the Hawaii Ironman, but it was no vacation! For my wife and kids, it was. But I was there racing. I always had a curiosity and respect for those battling for the overall win at the Hawaii Ironman Triathlon, but the times I spectated, I always stuck around until the official cut off to see everyone finish. Tearjerker stuff. That's why I was there in 1988 and again in 1989. I was searching. In 1998 I qualified and flew over there confidently, but I got smoked by a Navy Seal also paralyzed and although that's understandable, I hated it because I was sick, my bike wouldn't shift, and I had a bad day, but like those I saw finishing in the dark, I finished. The next two years racing the same Navy Seal I lost again and then in 2000, I finally didn't have any trouble, except a flat tire and I won. Finally! The inertia of all that training kept me healthy for almost another 10 years. Finally, too many airplanes, not the same exercise regimen, and not the same diet combined with age, I developed a pressure sore, which became infected and lead to the nightmare I had heard about years earlier. I spent 2 years barely sitting and a good 10 months on my stomach 24/7 in bed waiting for a good doctor who could put an end to it. He did, but it required 2 more months to get the surgery and another month post op before I could even sit up in bed in nearly a year. How did Jim Knaub escape that in all his years I thought? He didn't! At the lowest point I weighed 122lbs and questioned everything including living. After all, I had accomplished so much before and after my initial spinal cord injury (SCI) and now this? I was over it. But that idea of finishing crept back in. In training for motocross and then after motocross for a 5K on up to an Ironman, I always tried to finish on a good note. Fast and strong. I'd somehow figure out a way to find a little extra and do it! So, I thought, it's about as bad as it gets, others have it worse, so rather than fade to nothing with little ambition, I made the decision to get it together! I ignored all the, "haven't I suffered enough" and just tried to improve. For my wife, for the kids, for family, fans and people who had supported me for so many years. I couldn't give up. There were plenty of excuses and reasons, but I couldn't and believe me I was worn out. So, I'd sit up 5-minutes a day for a week, then 10, then 15 until 40 minutes. A final visit to the doctor and a green light! Walking again like I whined about when I first got hurt was a distant memory. I just wanted to be about to sit through a movie or go out to dinner. All I had been through already was enough evidence that I could make life fun and worth living again. But it would require my best - every day. That turned into training with and helping a younger kid who had been injured similarly to me to do the Ironman. That led to me thinking I'd like to head over to Hawaii and do another one, just to end on a good note. To finish strong and then who knows. So, in 2009 I did. I lead most of the day and with 10 miles to go in the marathon, this kid 13 years younger, also hurt racing motocross, the kid whom I had helped the same way Knaub helped me, pulled even and got a gap on me and I couldn't close it. I was bummed. But on the last hill into town with a few miles to go, knowing I was going to get 2nd, I stopped. I sat there looking at the sunset. Beautiful. The whole journey, spending my pre-injury honeymoon there in 1986 and thinking, I don't know how, but when I'm through racing motorcycles, I want to come over and do this race! Truth is, had I not been injured I'd have probably never qualified because I couldn't run fast enough. As that sunset slowly faded, I reminded myself, a couple years ago I was barely hanging on, so frail, so weak and unable to do the most basic things and yet here I am. That's something! And the kid beating me, well I had helped years earlier. Good for him. I coasted much of the way to the finish so happy that I was given a pass, grabbed hold of it and did the work, kept my mind from sinking into where it could easily go and instead, focused on what I could do. Then I heard the announcer, "David Bailey.

You are an Ironman!" Then I saw my wife, our son, my dad, and friends. I made it through so much hardship and doubt, and it all came pouring out at the same time. Some of the happiest tears of my life. I didn't care what place I got. Since there was nobody behind me, I sat there for 5-10 seconds thinking wow, I never thought I would be there again and couldn't imagine a reason to be there again so I soaked it all up appreciating there was even such a thing as that event that has changed lives. No wonder that event caught my attention in 1982. Who'd a thought I'd be there, the way I ended up there? The message of the Ironman for me was, "Keep Going!" You'll always be glad you did. If you don't, you'll always regret it.

ST: How has your experience of living without the ability to walk allowed you a different perspective on life?

I'm often asked about walking again or sent some article about some research or a clinical trial somewhere and somebody is walking again. For a few years I thought about it every day. Over the next decade or so I thought about it once in a while. But the truth is, I already walked for a quarter of a century. I won championships, world championships, traveled the world, met a great woman, have a family and 7 grandkids! Is walking really that important. At 62, I've noticed that a lot of people my age or older are looking for a place to sit down. What most don't say because it's not popular or perhaps too embarrassing to discuss, walking is last on the list. I'd like some stomach muscles. Maybe some bladder function or to have a cup of coffee and take a dump. Sexual function would've been nice. That took a hit and was tough to live without, especially knowing most other spinal cord injured victims are having fun and maybe even taking it for granted. But my inability to walk wasn't making my life a bummer. All those other things I lost were. Losing a good career racing so abruptly and the money I was starting to make, having my wife and best friend watch me suffer, having to figure out something else to do for a living that I'd probably never have chosen. That was hard. I was forced to focus on what all I had and did and experienced pre-injury and be thankful I had that. Post injury, with my limitations I was forced to figure things out and to really appreciate things like I never did because I was too busy, in a hurry, under pressure or worried about what was next. I came down to what Jim Knaub told me back in 1990. "Bailey, why walk when you can fly." When I was newly injured and still in the hospital, some people in my room were pointing at the TV, saying look! As I did, I saw a huge group of wheelchair racers in the Boston Marathon flying down a hill in the rain when one of them swerved, got up on two wheels, almost saved it, didn't and took out most of the filed at about 40mph! That was Jim Knaub. Six years later I was on the 2nd row of the starting line in the middle, right behind Jim and then flying down that same hill. Tragedy, comedy, to wow. Keep going. You never know. Here I am.

ST: Some victims of life-changing injury or illness offer that their lives are better, if not more interesting than if it would not have happened. Do you feel that way? Or would you rather have never gone through what you have?

Reflecting on my life's journey, there are some things I would like to have done. I wanted to race motorcycles in Europe in the 500cc World Championship. I thought it would be great to travel Europe with my wife, learn another language, maybe two and hopefully win the world championship over there. That had my interest, but I never got the chance. Racing here in America, I participated in or won more than I ever dreamed. I met Gina in 1984, traveled the world with her, thank God, and did and saw so much before I crashed … before things changed. It went about as good as it could go! I get stopped today by people, "We named our daughter after you. You were the best, my favorite, blah, blah." I'm not sure how much different it would've been had I never made it to Fresno for a nothing race and crashed and woke up to a new reality. I didn't like it one bit! None of it, but without the valleys, there are no mountaintops. It might've led me to too much time away from home and my wife, temptations or who knows. I could've just as easily messed up my life with all the freedoms, money, and time I had. This I do know. I did way more, saw and experienced way more than I thought I would've! From television to a magazine columnist, a coach, designer, an Ironman finisher, and a race across America finisher. Who would have thought? Not me. I thought my life was over when I ended up in a wheelchair and a couple of times I kind of wished it was. I've learned over the years that I'm only as strong as I need to be and whatever trouble comes my way, as much as I don't like it, there is a lesson in it and it's worth the trouble.

ST: How do you advise other spinal cord injury victims when you see them going through the same emotions that you suffered? Is that fulfilling or does it bring you a degree of nostalgic sadness?

A spinal cord injury is cruel. There are worse things, but it's devastating. And it's permanent. You don't rehab it and it's over. You wear it for the rest of your life. There are brief respites here and there. Maybe it's on a jet ski, or floating in a pool, but you can't ever get away from it. You don't stand up and walk down the road. Nothing else compares to the finality of it all. I witness it and hear it all the time. Parents are devastated because their son or daughter just crashed and is paralyzed. They'd give anything to get them out of it. To find a cure. Anything but life in a wheelchair! I listen and I understand, but what they don't know is what that can turn into. What direction it might take and how many people it can affect in a good way. I heard a friend say, hell maybe it came from you, "If the washing don't getcha, the rinsin' will." Things happen and there is nothing you can do, I tell them. But I think you'll be amazed. I think your child might surprise you.

ST: In many ways it seems that you didn't just "go through" rehab but your entire life, post-accident, is just one big rehabilitation process. Can you imagine that there may be a point in your life—if not achieved already—that you decide, "I'm not in rehab, I'm not "learning how to adapt to life in a chair" ... this is who I am until I die.

I didn't like the idea at first of anyone, even Jim Knaub telling me it's going to be fine. You'll adapt. You'll get used to it. How can I look at my wife and not want to just tackle her? How can I imagine being a dad and can't carry them around on my shoulders? Even though Jim Knaub was right about many things including what I could possibly do, I didn't want to hear it. But time has a way of changing your perspective. You do get used to it. You have to. You can fight it and be bummed and a drag for others or just move on and do your best. The Michael Jordan quote, "I missed 100% of the shots I didn't take" stands out. If I kept dwelling on being hurt, what was lost, I might never have said screw it, I'll give it a shot. I just played golf with my son and wife yesterday! I used to honk as I drove by a golf course or a range and think it was funny. Now, I hear somebody honk and think ... they'll learn!

Prescript: Between 1978 and 1980, fresh out of college with no plans or direction, I found my way into paramedic school and spent two years working on a box ambulance. Best and worse job I ever had. Made me grow up and hardened like war does. I spent a lot of time in fire stations working with fire fighters, in ERs working with ER docs and nurses and was amazed at their ability to process the obscene underbellies of the life we were all exposed to. In 1980, few people spoke openly about PTSD. Emotional trauma was just part of the job. Get over it or get out. It was only in crafting this tale based on a real call we rolled on that night John Lennon was shot, December 10th, 1980, that I realized men and women who work in emergency services are always and already in a state of rehabilitation, always seeking and finding ways to dodge and parry the horribleness that is part of their daily work. They don't "go into rehab." They ARE rehab.

Over Her, Over Me

> *"War cures all neurosis."*
>
> —Anna Freud

The call came in at 3:35 A.M. It's always around that time when the real fuckups come out. Why don't they disturb other people's lives during normal business hours? The P.D. routed the call after they'd sent a unit out on a noise disturbance complaint. When the officers arrived at the scene and poked around the apartment, they smelled smoke and called us.

Sometimes the lazy cops or the rookies or the guys who got their ass kicked in poker last week will call the fire department prematurely. Still, most of the calls like this are a tease, like a friend's wife who likes to flirt. We live for the ones that come in as a "fully involved, working fire," the sound of urgency straining through the consistent calm of dispatch. Dragging a charged two-inch hose into a Douglas fir and stucco-fueled hell, licking that bitch with a sweeping fog pattern, laughing at the top of your lungs; that's no job, that's a drug.

On this night though, we wouldn't get that jolt of watching flames spill through the roof and lick the sky like some giant tongue in search of its prey. No, this one was different. It might hold a place in our memories alongside the best working fires of our careers, but that place would be well sealed and unavailable to all but the ones who had to go there from time to time. God's chisel would not change that night.

It works like this.

The call comes in over the "George Orwell," our name for the loudspeaker, and wakes all of our asses up. There are twelve of us in this station: four on the pump, four on the ladder truck, two desk jockeys, the Captain and a Battalion Chief who wishes he was still pulling hose instead of pushing paper.

Two of us double as fire fighter/paramedics and respond to medical calls and structure fires in a box ambulance we call "the rig." I've never called it an ambulance. I suppose it's just a superstitious thing and all; like the way fighter pilots avoid using the word "crash."

I was on the rig that night and something in the air or on the ground or in between left me less than my Teflon self; the emotional landscape I'm used to where nothing sticks. Maybe it was the burritos that firefighter, Carter made for dinner, the argument I had with my wife before coming on shift or the two strings I'd broken on my guitar earlier that evening. It probably was nothing at all. But I didn't expect happy dreams.

We lay in bed, hoping for a quiet night unless it's something worth getting up for; something real ... that drug.

But we're jerked awake by "the George," recalled from wherever our minds had taken our bodies. Some of us pray a bit, if the early day has not been kind and we are so inclined, and then listen for the dispatcher to tell us which unlucky bastards have to climb out of a warm bed and go deal with the side of life God didn't spend enough time working on.

We don't all pray to the same God, but the presence of danger has a way of bringing you fully alive, frighteningly aware of things like the way dogs circle around their bed before lying down or the way a house always smells better when kids and fresh bread and cut wood is around. The presence of fear, even thimble amounts, will make you wonder how we all got here in the first place, trees and dogs included. When you're on shift, you look at life in full color, full time. There are no black and white images. You pay attention to everything, and you pray, hoping that your prayers don't just go out the widow behind the smoke of somebody's cigarette.

And on this night, this December 10th, the year nineteen hundred and eighty, miserable *can't make up its mind* weather outside, not raining, not dry, more like the clouds were dripping a cold sweat, George Orwell sent the pumper and the rig on account of the smoke.

I whispered a little "Thank you," not really caring to who it was directed, snickered at the thought of Captain and Larry and Cala and Carter having to put on cold, clammy turn-outs, probably still wet from that practice hose lay we did before dinner, and go chase some hokey, "smell-of- smoke," bullshit call. I know that Carter is hoping the cops will get in the building, find nothing more than burnt spaghetti noodles left on the stove and turn them around. But it ain't going to happen. My stomach does something, and I lay there for a few seconds listening to the rain and the men.

Nobody complains about it in front of Captain either. He cuts us a lot of slack, and it seems he has always known what we know now. We save the wimpy complaints for each other while washing the trucks or drinking beer after work. Some of the guys will dump on a new girlfriend who might not understand what we do but the wives, well, they mostly have had a guts-full and tell us that if we don't like it, we can quit it. But that isn't likely, knowing in our hearts there ain't a better job when you pull someone's ass out of trouble or get dealt a quiet shift and just work around the station, relaxing after five with a Scrabble game or a few songs out on the porch; just watching the rest of the nine to fivers head home to their wives and their kids and their homes.

Sometimes I wish I was one of them, knowing that when they went to sleep, chances were slim to none some old man would be calling them up to come and put him back in bed because his legs were all stoved up.

But when I am getting off work in the morning, nothing planned for the day, a full night's sleep behind me, and I see that same guy heading to his office to drive a desk all day, well, I'm not in too big a hurry to switch lives.

The clock on the wall says 3:36 A.M., four more hours until I can be home, a bit later if I stop at Moonshiner's for some eggs and a game of pool if I see a truck or two, I know in the dirt lot.

Dammit all, though. No sooner than my head falls back into the pillow, the dispatch comes on again and says for Medevac 12 to respond with the pump. "Possible woman down," I catch, while scribbling down the address in case we get split up from the fire truck.

It's my turn to drive this shift and my partner, Tommy Willard, a fresh, young kid right out of the academy who's only working his second go-around, is still wrestling with his helmet in the corner as I fire up the rig and chase the pump out the big bay door into the moonless night.

"C'mon Probie," I goad him, "You ain't gonna' need that skid lid with me at the wheel." Tommy jumps in, slams the door just before it gets ripped off the rig by the station wall and tells me he only wears it "on account of he don't want to be seen with a guy as ugly as me." The kid still on probation has balls. I like him a lot.

We drive through the dark, empty night, silent in our thoughts, the occasional siren used only to keep night owls honest. There's a pissy rain keeping even the hard-core drunks holed up in some place of their own making. I am awake now, alive and watching the strobe lights of the big pumper truck in front of us reflect off the dampened avenues. The city's asphalt street-veins are deserted except for a couple of red trucks and a half dozen grown men and women who got lucky enough or stupid enough to find them living out the fantasy of many young boys. I get a strong sense of ownership at times like this; like the well-being of this little town sort of belongs to me and the crew. I know any one of us could mess up bad in a heartbeat. But the responsibility doesn't scare me, and we are as fitting to the job as bark to a tree. We share meals and stories and lies and truths.

I look over at Tommy as he's picking up the mic to go 10-97 (arrived on scene), a look of thinly veiled anticipation in his eyes and I wonder if he will have the same feeling when he is as old as me, has seen what I have seen, and has dealt with the ambiguity behind it all. Soon enough he'll realize that human trauma is greedy. It deserves all of our attention.

3:42 A.M.

We park the rig beside the pump, grab the med bag, 02 bottles, de-fib machine and haul ass up the stairs just behind Captain, Larry and Cala. Carter is the engineer, so he stays with the pump panel. He's okay with that. He has a couple of kids now.

The probie trips on the first step and I don't even think about laughing. Until we do our job and clear the scene, nothing's funny, not on the inside nor the outside. We aren't hired to play God, but we ain't selling stocks and bonds either. I used to feel things. Now I don't feel much at all. And I'm better at my job because of that fact, just keeping my empathy wrapped up cellophane tight, an old sandwich setting in the back of the fridge. Maybe you'll get around to eating it before it goes bad on you.

P.D. has finally gotten the locked door pried open and we all enter the mysterious apartment and source of the loud music and smoke. We go in as a tribe more than a group, a collection of cogs in a machine, one that has the ability to alter some natural law of living and dying. But the only thing I know for sure is that I won't stand for people going and getting hurt or suffering needlessly on *my* shift, even if I don't feel much of anything about it later.

Captain has a strange sense of forecast—he's seen it many times before in his duty with this city. He's the kind of man who will leave a mark on the world, unlike most of the ones you meet who just get marked up.

Something's not right, his eyes and gestures tell me.

Waving the others back, he motions for me to come along, confident in our time and years. Not much gets through the veneer that this job has given me cause to grow. He turns slow as a dime store Indian and asks directly, "You're a Beatles fan, aren't you?"

3:48 A.M., 3:50 tops. I put the thought of the huevos rancheros at Shiner's out of my mind and focus my light on Captain's big, yellow-coated back as I follow him down the long smoky hall. "NFD" it says, Nashville Fire Department. Or NO Fucking Dying. He's not really human at times like this, but part predator and part angel. If he ever got killed, I think I might go ahead and pray to him too.

We reach the closed bedroom door and can clearly hear a John Lennon song through the walls, "*Instant karma's gonna' come and get you ...*" But what almost

51

knocks me off my feet is the smoky scent that initiated this run. It is not the familiar smell of burning wood or plastic or clothes or even the unmistakable stench of crispy bodies. It is the sickly-sweet stench of too many cheap candles. I've seen it before, felt it, and wondered about it at hippie weddings, weirdo funerals, and Catholic churches where you get a year of credit in Purgatory for each cheap little blue candle that you pay to light.

Cap nudges the door open far enough for us to get a glimpse of what it is that will leave another fucked up imprint on our minds; not if, but a question of degree. I had called the candles right. There must have been dozens of them all lit up in shapes and sizes, pyramids, globes, long skinny cylinders, headstone masts from a hundred sunken ships illuminating a no man's land between this life and the one after. Heck, there over on the chest of drawers next to the stereo was a candle shaped like Mickey Mouse, a glowing red, yellow and blue flame between his wax ears. Full color, full time.

At the foot of the bed was a shitty 13-inch TV, the screen showing the snow pattern that used to come after the 11:00 News was over and before cable brought you people trying to sell worthless crap that you wouldn't buy from a neighbor at his garage sale just to be nice. On one wall hung a suggestive, stylistic poster of a man and women, framed together like two pieces of puzzle, he on top, she on the bottom, naked on the bed. It was photographed in black and white, but I could have made it color by blinking my eyes.

And there, lying wonderfully serene in the middle of her bed, was a majestic young lady dressed in bell bottom Levi's and a lavender flannel pajama top. Her long blond hair straight, thick and shiny in front, matted wet and red, molded to the pillow in the back. She seemed like she would have been easy to love. And though I fought the emotion, I hated her for that.

It was then, as the old cassette player switched to, "In My Life" and I heard the words, "with lovers and friends I still can recall", that I looked around the room and realized that we were in some type of Lennon shrine.

I stood over her, her eyes still wide in search of some meaning to it all. But I still had to verify the condition, document the diagnosis, and get "permission" from the hospital not to work her up. When someone opts to eat a single .44 caliber bullet for dinner, there just isn't a lot you can do for them.

I got the hospital on the radio, trying not to look as the Captain took off his glove and closed her eyes with his rough, weathered hand. Larry, a regular hose man from southern Nebraska and the best bass fisherman among us, walked down the hallway after having scoped out the rest of the apartment. He was humming Dylan's "Lay Lady Lay" and when he peered into the bedroom and saw the Cap with his big mitts on the girl's face, he spoke the line, "his clothes are dirty, but his hands are clean." The words left his mouth without malice, nor thought, nor intent. Stuff like that comes out. It just does. You don't even think about it at the time.

I hung up the phone and Cap pulled the sheet over her face. I tried not to but still, I told him what he already knew, but that I needed to say, "There's no excuse, no damn rhyme or reason. It's as simple as that. Bitch had to go and die on our shift."

Like I said, some private transactions with the ordinary unlucky, on a regular shift.

And as I turned away to leave the room, the edge of my coat knocked over a candle, dousing a single flame and spilling hot wax onto my grimy, black rubber boots. Oddly, grotesquely, secretly, I admired her courage, disdained her cowardice, wished I could have known her in another life and felt the heat from the warm wax.

Captain came over and looked at me, his eyes asking if I was all right.

"Life's an accident but death ain't," he said and went outside to have a cigarette.

I just nodded, ignoring the coroner's arrival and asked Tommy to drive the rig while I sat in the cab on the way back to the station. Watching the sun trying to rise and break through the passing front, dancing reds and yellows peering through the grays, I told myself that this must be the way with firefighters and medics and cops and corpsmen: process the emotion and move on. You don't think about a young child's love for his pet puppy when you are dragging his little body out of a burning building. Caring will make you soft, I told myself. Yep. Thinking will ruin you.

I asked Tommy if he believed in God.

"On the good days," he told me. Not an unexpected reply.

"You?" he asked, pulling into the station driveway.

53

"Oh yeah," I whispered, "Because it's amazing how much blood can come out of one little body."

We walked back inside just as the morning news was coming on. Well past 6:00 A.M. now. A hair-sprayed talking head was reporting on last night's murder of John Lennon outside his Manhattan apartment building. The young crew was crowded around the TV set, making referenced jokes about the call last night. Just another defense mechanism, I thought. Let it go. How could they have known what John Lennon meant to his fans, to the world, to the girl last night?

Tommy, who was four years old when the Beatles first came to JFK Airport, was coming up with the best lines, building his own protective layer, one cynical crack at a time. Yep, that's the way with firefighters—risk it, defy it, Betty's Crocker or Dante's fucking hell. Do everything humanly possible to drown Darwinism with 5,000 gallons per minute from a charged hose or 1000cc of Ringer's Lactate direct I.V. Later on, diffuse it all with laughter; just give it away.

God, Allah, the Great Spirit, fucking Santa Claus ... we aren't any of these guys. Hell, we aren't even docs. Not on this night. Not ever. We're just firemen, veterans of a different kind of war.

I sat in front of my locker and took off my turnouts, trying not to look at the melted wax on my boot. Tommy walked in and asked me if I wanted to get some breakfast when we got off shift in a few minutes. My eyes, filling with tears now, looked up at Tommy and gave him his answer. He stared at the floor, not quite confused, not quite embarrassed and tried to say something. But no sound came from his mouth.

I dragged my sleeve across my face, got up and headed out to my truck. Passing the Battalion Chief in his office, it was 7:30 A.M., twenty-four hours since I started this shift. Nothing's different, I lied, just a day in life, another collision of empathy and emptiness.

"Don't forget to do your Patient Run Report before you leave. Numbers got to be right."

Sure Chief, I thought, numbers have to be right. Sometimes patients, sometimes victims.

Always numbers.

Always human.

The sun was fully operational now, the bright colors reflecting off the panes of my truck's windshield as if the glass itself were on fire. Reaching first for the bottle of Jack Daniels under the seat and then for my old Martin acoustic behind the cab, I swallowed hard and wondered if I could still play it. Tears were streaming down my cheeks, salty raindrops onto a spruce body, I was exposed in the morning's light, a cracked shell lying on the wet tarmac, the truth exploding out of my gut like a running dog unleashed.

I sat on the truck's tailgate, a street fight happening inside my heart and watched as my fingers went right for the rosewood neck, hitting the frets slowly but accurately: D, F#mi, Em7, A and then A7, just like the first day I taught myself the song several lifetimes ago. I mouthed the words to myself, "*Pools of sorrow, waves of joy are drifting through my open mind …*," took a long pull on the bottle, setting it down next to the guitar, knowing they deserved each other.

When I looked up, Captain was lumbering out to his own truck, a big duffel bag full of firefighter stuff slung over one shoulder, just enough teeth showing in his smile to let me know that he knew and that he cared as much as he was able.

Cap set the bag down next to my rusted tailgate and sat down on it. He was carrying a bag like we all do; dirty t-shirts, a couple of magazines on fishing, hunting or cars, a Tupperware bowl that held cookies from yesterday morning, a few tapes, maybe a Bible, maybe this month's centerfold. Everything smelled of smoke. Mostly the Bibles. A lot of important things aren't easily cleaned.

I passed him the bottle, but he shook his head and grunted, reaching instead for the guitar, inspecting it like he was considering a delicate piece of art. Then he played one strange chord way up on the neck, reached up to the gold tuners and gave the low E a gentle twist, altering the sound in a way few could tell.

"Flatten the low E string just a tad. Gives that song a raw sound and fills out the bottom some."

And then he got up to leave, passing back my axe as he would a newborn.

Walking away, he stopped, turned just slightly, enough so I could hear him but not see his face and said in a voice softer than I remembered him owning, "Not much left to kill or die for; nope, not too much left at all."

"Well," I chocked back a reply, "If there is I reckon we'll see it first."

"Yep, I imagine we well," he said. "See ya tomorrow, huh," not asking but confirming, and threw his duffel bag in the back of his truck.

Everything else could stay here at the station.

Prescript: Anyone who has ever lost a favorite domestic animal has suffered the vagaries of loss; has been thrown suddenly into a dark state of confusion. The return to normalcy can take months or years. There is just something about losing a good dog. In some ways, I'd rather lose a human acquaintance than my mans-best-friend. That will sound harsh if you're not a dog person. The rehabilitation from losing a fellow mammal—especially if they have slept in your bed for years—is never easy. I know it's a cliché but the only healer I know is time. The notion of rehabilitation here extends to WHY we mourn the loss of an animal. It must range from the overly dramatic "any loss of one of God's creatures is a tragedy" to the more practical "that animal never judged me like people do" to the brutally honest "I just miss my friend." My family and I have rehabilitated from the loss of our dog and have enjoyed the steady brilliance of several replacements who have met the task. To this day though, I still think about my dog Molly.

Life Be Proud

> *"And if you gaze for long into an abyss,*
> *the abyss gazes also into you."*
> —Frederick Nietzsche

> *"A dog's short life is God's cruel trick."*
> —Unknown

I'm just driving around digging holes in every dry creek bed and big, open field that I come across. It's past midnight and in the back of my truck are two shovels, a pair of gloves, and a large green tarp. I'm digging holes because it's the only thing I can think of doing right now. I need a grave, but truth be known, the feel of shoveling into earth is primal—I need to punish myself as well.

My twelve-year-old son sits next to me, steadily as a battle-worn veteran. "It's not your fault dad. The poison was way up high in some neighbor's wood pile. Someone must've knocked it down." He's right, I try to convince myself, but I have to feel the pain of remorse, wallow in the guilt until some sad wisdom of compromise finally gains a rational foot hold. I won't dig potential graves all night long, but I might hemorrhage in other ways for months to come.

It took me thirty years to find the perfect dog: gentle with a strong spirit, inquisitive but compliant, friendly yet protective, as loyal as a bark to tree. And now she lay inside a green tarp in the back of my truck, her lithe and limber six-year-old legs stiffening with each new hole I dig, deeper and wider to accommodate, in sync with the daggered reality that d come the next morning. I'd call out her name in the pre-dawn chill to go run ... and then I'd remember.

"Dad, maybe we'd just better take her home and call some place in the morning that does this kinda' stuff."

"No, we can bury her right. That the least I can do for ...," then I'd wipe my dirty sweatshirt across my eyes and fish the back roads of my brain for the smallest reconciliation of peace.

I'd been sitting in a chair at the university when I heard the news from my wife—*I think something is seriously wrong with Molly,* she pushed the air out of her chest and into the phone. *I think she might be even ... dead.*

Everything went out from underneath me, the chair, my office floor, the earth. And now there was no real estate left for me to put her memory into.

I'm not a pure animal lover. That makes it worse, because when you find one you like, you latch on to it to prove to yourself that you aren't a callous asshole. The dog knows that and all the while you think you're training them, they're teaching you. Dogs know more than we ever give them credit for. Molly knew she was dying a full day before she laid down on the back deck in the sun, careful to lay her head facing away from the house so that the kids wouldn't have to see her before my wife came home and covered her up.

The morning, she died, she had the saddest look of any living creature I'd ever seen. Her eyes were trying to capture us, pull us inside of her so that we could see the damage and pain of the poison; the way it must've been eating her alive, one organ at a time. It was a soundless scream for help, "I'd love to go running with you mom but I'm dying, and it hurts like hell. You go ahead." And as always, I was late for something; just waved through the window as my wife ran her hand through her fur a few times and checked on her uneaten food while I left them—one to come back to and cry with, the other forever.

There were other signs that we missed: the way she walked a dead man's walk, head down, eyes seeking purchase on anybody who could help, tail flat and somber.

I didn't arrange her birth; didn't even raise her from a pup. She was a "pound dog," the best kind. Some other jerk missed the wholeness in her spirit while complaining that she couldn't point or that she'd dug holes in his putting green lawn. I brought her home and we became kin. We respected each other.

"Hey mom," the kids might've said, "Molly looks sick." She might've barked or growled or thrown up blood or lied down in the middle of the room and refused to move. A lot of things might've happened. I might've thought better about it even knowing that rat poison lived on my street. Maybe even in my yard. Death … not if but when? Would of, should of … shit. Life is a choice, I thought, not hastily. Death isn't.

But in a gallant and gracious death as this, when one of God's creatures cannot heal themselves and then go off into the forest to die alone rather than bother the clan, they are mythologized in the hearts of those who might've done something. In cultural history passed down through oral tradition, campfire tales and classroom textbooks, they become legend. The Hero's Journey cannot belong only to the world of men.

Thirty years and I had the perfect dog in the back of my truck, cold and stiff, waiting for the animal shelter to open up in the morning so I could deliver my legend. They'll tell me it's a shame, she had a good home for a while, a better life than many animals, but none of that will register. I will be thinking of how she died, how she must've suffered. I will forever be thinking of her eyes. And wondering why I could not learn to read them; wondering if I could foresee the silent hopeful scream in those that might follow. Right then, I heard her body slide across the plastic bed liner and bump into the walls of the truck bed.

I've watched enough death in my life. I've seen men fight it all the way to their last gasp, and beyond. Right out of college I worked for a period as a paramedic in a big city, a young man doing a hard job. I was stationed at an inner-city fire station. There were days when I felt like an innocent medic tossed into the jungles of

Southeast Asia. Only we had real docs on the phone and could be at a good hospital in 10 minutes. But when death comes knocking, the sound of its resonating steps, the sound has a kind of universality you might only find when something is born.

"That's it," my young paramedic partner would say after rolling up on an obvious DOA. And we'd call the hospital, get clearance to cease patient care and shut their eyes for them, just like in the movies. But even under the white sheet, I could see tiny muscle twitches, little noises crying out of their mouths.

"Just a natural post-mortem physiological reaction," the doctors had told us in school, "the body's way of cooling down." But I didn't believe it. I was already invested in the legends, way too superstitious or too spiritual to be doing that job. So, I quit. And got myself a dog. Dogs would die of old age while sleeping next to the warm fire and dreaming of when they knew how to catch a Frisbee in midair only five years ago. I could handle that.

===

Three weeks later, I was better about forgetting, but I'm also quicker to remember. What I'm feeling is that I miss my dog, but I begin to forget the little things, like the way she'd chase her own shadow or stop just before catching a rabbit, as if to say, "Be more careful. I won't eat you, but others will."

Forgetting—it's the mind's way of dealing with loss—to dole it out in small palatable bites, like liver to a child. What has sharpened in focus, though, is the reality of what I remember, and now swallow as reconstituted truth: it's that Molly, the Brittany spaniel, just another man's dead dog to some, represented what courage and grace could be found in death. She had joined her life and her death, seamlessly, suffering without asking, hurting but giving back, moving out to the edge of the long, dark neighborhood forest, and dying alone because she could not heal herself. And those around her who loved her without even knowing it, who on a normal day would have her with them, had meetings to attend. Life can get in the way of living sometimes.

Animals are tough like kids are tough. It stems from their innocence. When they hurt, they don't look for someone to blame or to sue; they look for comfort and wait for it to pass. Kids grow into adults and are subjected to society's jagged barbs that morph into jingoistic ambivalence. Animals don't read the papers or buy new shoes when they feel bad. They die the way they are born, innocent and wanting to please. And their deaths remind us of how far we have become removed from the purity of youth, begging the question, "What the hell *happened* to me?"

There are good people who die well every day. And there are mean, vicious animals that should be put to sleep. The generalizations are fair and arguable at the same time. But when a good man or a good dog dies, they take with them a part of the living, leaving all that they gave to better the human condition. What Molly took with her was the unconditional love found more often in good dogs than even in good humans. What she left was the hope that it can still exist, that humans still have a chance to catch up.

But sometimes it takes the worst to bring out our best. Like war or tragedy.

They say that many humans lose 21 to 23 grams of weight at the exact moment they die. You couldn't label it as evidence of souls, but it can be comforting though, when wrestling with your own mortality; the idea that a part of you, maybe the best part or maybe the only part, goes somewhere else. Life-transition is doable. Death seems awfully permanent.

And tragedy temporary.

That night as I carried her around the open field looking for a proper resting place, she became heavier, though my memory is that of her feeling lighter the next day. The scales of love and hope could never balance each other; the fluidity and interdependence just too strong for even a momentary equilibrium.

I am haunted by those dying eyes of my dog, cursed to remember so I won't forget. On some early morning runs, my breath coming out like white smoke signals, I have the courage to run alone, to go forth in an attempt to concretize and finally bury what I feel about the way people love, the way they die, and the inseparable connection between the two. But as soon as I create the answer, I must erase it; the pain of associated memory coming back up in bites too large to swallow in one meal.

This too, is the way men think of each other in war. After a while, it's not about nations or battles or even going home. It's about your buddy—staying alive because you'll let him down if you get killed. Any soldier will tell you that. When things get heavy, fuck patriotism. You don't go and get shot because you will disappoint your pals.

I imagine Molly was disappointed that she'd let me down by dying.

And as the sun burns one day into the next, memories of that simple dog-love reshape the past, and then file the edges off the pain and the unvanquished death into a kind of razor's edge of admiration. I think finally, indelibly, that if I do know but one thing about my rehabilitation from the fear of dying, it is this: whether you're talking about good or evil, humans or dogs, war or peace, it begins inside, travels to the eyes and ends up in the world.

And there it stays. Living.

Prescript: I'm not afraid of many things but somewhere I have this latent fear of being wrongfully accused of a crime, convicted, and sent off to prison. Apparently, it happens more than we hear about. But I've never been to jail, and I'd like to think my life will end with my streak intact. I have a few friends and acquaintances who have done some time. The majority are misdemeanors for things like DUI and petty theft. But a few, as chronicled below, are convicted felons and spent over a year behind bars or in detention camps. Speaking with them over the years revealed vastly different ideas on how they returned and "healed" if I can use that word, from their incarceration.

The Big House

There are currently thirty-four prisons in the state of California housing somewhere between ninety and one hundred thousand inmates. The median age of inmates is increasing as is the cost (estimated at $125,000 in 2025) to keep them behind bars. Nearly one third of the prisons and "camps" operate over suggested capacity. And while the trend over the last few years is a slow reduction in the California prison population, several prisons are closed each year. Assault, robbery, and weapons charges count for more than fifty percent of the convictions each year. According to the National Institute on Drug Abuse, one in five are jailed for illegal substance trafficking.

The data on how long a convicted felon serves time appears relative to the severity of the crime, their behavior while incarcerated, the skill of their lawyer, and inherent politics of their parole board. Sometimes what we see in films, TV, and news sources reflect an accurate portrayal of time behind bars. But many times, it is sensationalized if not false. A friend of mine, let's call him Harry, refers to this as the "Alcatraz Effect" and enjoys the pathetic fallacy of high-tech escapes as portrayed in popular culture. Harry did three and one-half years for involuntary manslaughter.

Harry is not my only friend who did time in jail or the "Big House." Others were incarcerated for DUIs, drug possession, and financial crimes. While none did long or hard times, all of them returned to society with a record and a memory of lost freedom. With new kinds of fear and nightmares. With an appreciation for the simple pleasures like turning the channel on your TV or taking a piss on the side of the trail while hiking in the woods.

In a collection of pieced-together notes and memories from conversations with these former inmates, I offer the responses below to my ranging questions about rehabilitation or what Morgan Freeman's character in the 1994 film, Shawshank Redemption, calls "just a made-up word. A politician's word so that young fellows like yourself can wear a suit and tie and have a job." But Freeman's character, Ellis Boyd Redding, challenges us to consider the term as it applies to the many and varied aspects of rehabilitating oneself after being convicted of a crime and serving time behind bar. For much of the 80s, 90s, and 2000s the recidivism rate in California was just below fifty percent. And while that number has inched slightly lower in recent years, it still reminds us that way too many people find themselves back in jail again and again. Rehabbing from jail is a complicated and harrowing issue. And I certainly don't pretend to know much about it.

Perhaps my contacts can shed some light. Because none of the participants wanted to be identified for fear of profiling (something telling in that fact), we'll call them Harry, Mary, and Tom. Each had their own memories about their return to society. I can't say that one approach or strategy or behavioral type was better than another but I'm sure there was some bearing. Being in jail or prison must be tough. Getting out could also be considered a challenge.

===

ST: You did your time for your crime. What do you remember most as you think about your time in 'rehab' from prison?

Harry: It was mostly the simple things I both enjoyed and struggled with. Like shopping for food, deciding where to buy gas for my car, and deciding when to fall asleep. In jail and prison, you lose a lot of privileges, but you come to fall into the rhythm of what is decided for you. That and having to tell people where I'd been. Imagine. "So, what you been up to, Bro?" "Ah, just sitting in the big house for running over a guy."

ST: Was the honesty of your incarceration a real struggle or did it eventually become part of your return to a normal life?

Harry: What's a "normal life" anymore? I've seen crazier things just driving around town than what I saw in prison. But yeah, at first it was hard to come to grips with the fact I was a convicted felon. And that label wasn't goin' away. I lost a lot of friends, but I made new ones; you know ... friends in low places, and I became tighter with the ones who stuck with me. After a while, maybe two or three years back on the streets, the conviction and label became a part of my history and thus, a part of who I was. I didn't like; wished I could erase the whole episode that night. Wished I hadn't tried to race that guy in the Camaro. Wished someone hadn't fukin' died. But it did and a big part of my rehabilitation was coming to accept my crime and its consequences.

ST: I've heard that in some strange way, the return to normal begins when you're convicted, and your sentence begins. Any thoughts on that?

Harry: I can see that. Jail changes people, even those overnight DUI cats who've never seen that part of society. Going to jail or prison for any length of time can reset a big part of your psyche. You're scared to shit at first but then you start to get used to being on edge all the time. And maybe if you're lucky, you start to realize the gravity of your position and know in your heart of hearts you don't ever want to come back here once you get out. So, whatever fucked up part of your personality landed you behind bars, you start to work on as soon and they slam that metal door.

ST: After you got out and started to find your way back to a more regular life, was there anything you'd do differently?

Harry: Well, I only did three and one-half years so not a lot of things had really changed. But I tried to rush back into my old life, tried to make up for lost time. In hindsight, I shoulda' chilled a bit and slowly found my way back. I really didn't have much support or counseling. But I'd tell that to the guys getting out now; take your time, appreciate your freedom. And remember the mistakes that put you there. For me, I stopped drinking and for at least a year, I wouldn't drive a car. Even now, years later, I see people leaving the restaurants and I can tell they've had a drink or three and when they get in their cars I want to reach in and grab their keys and throw them into the bushes. But I guess the main thing I'd wish I'd done was join a support group of a bunch of ex-cons. At the time, it didn't sound like a good idea. I was sick of dealing with guys who weren't exactly pillars of society. But now, when

I meet a fellow ex-con, we share something. Sometimes it's good. Sometimes it's bad. But it's always a reminder.

=====

ST: Mary, you did eighteen months for a financial crime at a low security prison. How do you think your rehabilitation was different from someone who did harder time?

Mary: Well, to be honest, I don't think you can compare them. I mean, a lot of these people are hardened criminals with long records. Maybe that's why their return to society isn't as complete. They can't adjust to a life without crime.

ST: That seems a bit of a totalizing statement. Can you consider that returning from having stolen millions of dollars from others or selling drugs for profit might share some similarities in the rehab process?

Mary: Corporate crime has been part of our national pastime since the Industrial Revolution. Taking money from others who basically "allow" you to take it is different than crimes where someone gets hurt. Hey, welcome to capitalism.

ST: If I'm hearing you correct, you feel that the victims of financial theft are different than say, assault and battery or murder. And by extension, you feel that rehabilitation is different.

Mary: I was part of a big machine that got caught. Okay, people lost a lot of money. But I'm not sure how my incarceration should be considered on the same level as someone who robs you at gunpoint.

ST: I hope that you don't mind me asking but do you feel sorry for what happened?

Mary: Of course I do, and I think I'm a better person for having been in a camp. I do hate to call it jail. And I wouldn't do what I did again. But I paid the price and, in some ways, because there were others around me who only got probation or a fine, I feel that I'm a victim as well.

ST: *Was there anything that the legal system did or did not do that effected your uh, "rehabilitation"?*

Mary: I went through all sorts of interviews but I always felt like the people were trying to figure out how we stole money so they could catch the next group who understand how to work the system and make money off people who just don't pay enough attention to their assets. I would've liked someone to be more empathetic to me and dug a bit deeper into why I chose that path; why even now, I probably don't feel as bad for the victims as I should.

=====

ST: *Tom, you did two and one-half years of a four-year sentence for assault with a deadly weapon. And general thoughts on your rehabilitation after prison?*

Tom: Ha! Yeah, I got a lot of thoughts. But the main thing is that the guy deserved it. That was a long time ago and even though I was young and stupid, I'm pretty sure I'd do it again. I mean, given the same circumstances.

ST: *Do you feel that your remorse or lack thereof, had anything to do with the way you successfully returned to society?*

Tom: Well, I wasn't ever completely removed from the real world when I was in prison. Family and friends came to visit, I studied, learned a lot. Followed the day-to-day happenings when we could get on the internet. And two and a half years isn't like doing twenty. But my crime was—in my head at the time—justified. So, yeah, while I feel like the legal system failed me in some ways, my "rehab" was acceptable.

ST: *Were you ever scared in prison?*

Tom: Hell, everyone is scared. If they tell you they're not, they're lying. But to be honest, I was still scared when I got out. They have the three strikes law in California and even after one felony, you have to be really careful you don't find yourself in a situation, the wrong place at the wrong time, which can land you back behind bars.

ST: So, is that law or others like it a positive thing for rehabilitation after jail?

Tom: It certainly is a motivator. But think about this. The majority of guys in prison for violent crimes at the federal level grew up on the wrong side of the tracks. A lot of them had to fight and steal and lie just to survive. And when they get out, they ain't going back to some goddamn Ozzie and Harriet cul-de-sac. It's a vicious cycle that's hard to break. If you're socialized in a street gang environment from a young age, that physical part of your adult life doesn't die easily.

ST: That might explain the high levels of recidivism. But still, I wonder if you can suggest any approaches or strategies that might help people as they try to reimagine a new, crime-free life?

Tom: The rules on the inside are different than the ones on the outside. If you're behind bars for even a few months or a year, you learn the official and unofficial rules. But then you're released, and you have to adapt. Inside, for example, you can make up a lot of shit and everyone knows you're lying but they don't care so long as it's creative and interesting. Outside, people expect you to tell the truth, especially in legal situations. The parole board and the so-called counselors might know of the dirty little secrets to adapting well but they can't teach you these. The best place to go for rehab advice is a support group of ex-cons.

ST: Was there a single moment after you got out that you felt you were going to be okay? That you could put your time in prison behind you?

Tom: You never put that time completely behind you. And maybe that's a good thing ... to remember. But yeah, there was a time; I ran into an old friend I hadn't seen in many years. He asked me what I'd been up to and I told him I'd been in the Big House. He laughed and said, "No really, what you been doing?" And I said no really, I've been in prison for almost three years for almost killing a guy. He sort of took a step back and looked at me curiously. And after a moment of uncomfortable silence he said, "Well, I'm sure he deserved it" and asked if I needed help with anything. I told him he'd just given me what I needed.

SECTION 2:

THE REHAB OF INJURY, ILLNESS, DISEASE

Introduction

When we think of rehabilitation, we often think of recovery from injury, illness, and debilitating disease. The benchmark programs for drug and alcohol rehab, the return from a bout with cancer or AIDS, the struggle to overcome clinical depression, and the nerve damage from a horrific crash. Loss of limb, sight, hearing, and speech. These are sampled elements of loss and fear that inhabit our negative core. We secretly hope that we are bypassed when the Hobgobs of broken bodies cast their spell. And then it happens. Our illnesses might be visible, or they might not. When in the fall of 1999, I lost 70% of my vision in my left eye due to a retinal vein occlusion, my 83-year-old mother, who had buried two husbands and faced mounting health issues, looked at me and said, "I don't see anything wrong with your eye. Besides, you have another one. Get over it."

And she was right.

We've all heard stories about a distant Uncle that never smoked or drank, he exercised, practiced yoga, meditation, and aromatherapy, ate only organic garlic and died when a truck delivering meat byproducts careened off the road and squashed him on his morning jog. Or the distant cousin who died peacefully overweight with a bottle of Jack Daniels in her hand at 97 years old.

My friend Yoni, a wicked smart and retired anesthesiologist, reminded me that as a male, if you live long enough, the chances of dying of prostate cancer increase exponentially. Hell, if he's right and I live to 100 years old and that shit finally gets me, well, I will have died old and satisfied.

We can do a lot to reduce our chances of disease and accident but at some point, the Fates win. Shit happens.

But here's the point. How we rehab from those challenges nearly defines us. Reminds us of who we are and why we were here. These stories help us to negotiate the vagaries of injury, illness, and disease when they come knocking.

Prescript: The essay below was written over twenty years ago when basal cell carcinoma took hostage to the tip of my nose. As the repair healed and the scar faded, I came to look at elective surgery in a new light; supportive of women and men who choose to have parts of their body altered. The nose, the eyes, the buttocks, the breasts … all are a key element to one's outward appearance and thus their sense of confidence, if not how they hold themselves up against a judgmental world. There is an understudied aspect of rehabilitation when a person—whether due to injury or illness or elective—returns from surgery that alters their looks. How we present to the world is often a reflection on how we feel about ourselves inside. I don't think anyone is immune. From the sixteen-year-old who notices a pimple on his nose right before a first date, to individuals who lose a limb; there is a need for resiliency and adaptation that is hard to teach and at times … even harder to learn.

Crooked Timber

> *"This face is all I have, worn and lived in;*
> *the lines around my eyes my old friends."*
>
> —Willie Nelson

I asked the nurse if she ever got used to the smell of burning flesh. She looked away from me and spoke through the white surgical mask, the same kind I had used to paint the bathroom the weekend before.

"Sure, you just don't notice it after a while."

Notice *what*, I thought, the smell, or the act of burning someone's flesh itself?

She must have sensed my confusion because she forced an awkward laugh, covering some deeper thought by making light of a serious situation. I'm sure she knew I was hiding behind a thin layer of macho veneer; this stable woman who cauterized each small blood vessel as the surgeon sliced away another layer of my face. She knew. They always do. It's their job.

My job was to be "okay" with the operation the docs were about to perform. Regardless of the outcome, whether a tiny snaking scar or Elephant Man, I needed to be ready.

I wasn't.

Cynicism is a bad thing. And I was cynical about plastic surgery, a term that isn't as apparent or descriptive as its semantic partners, "reconstructive" and "cosmetic." Vain men and women standing in line, I thought, paying huge sums of money for what is known as elective surgery (you choose to have it—there is no real medical need). Flip through the pages in the office, order off the menu. You want pouty lips, smooth cheeks, a thinner waist, thicker calves, high-beam boobs? The before/after pictures are always convincing.

But I'm a guy. Men can get away with crow's feet around the eyes and a few jagged lines left over from a motorcycle crash or an old football injury. Women *need* to look half their age. It says so right there on the cover of *Redbook, Cosmo*, and *Women's Day*. Forty-year-old guys who model underwear are considered rugged and must've been a famous jock at one time or another. Forty-year-old women do ads for estrogen supplementation.

Yeah, I was a real righteous cat. I may have appreciated the outline, if not the sculpture of augmented breasts (you really can't say "fake tits" anymore), but when I felt them, I was taken back to my days on the beach, shoveling jelly fish into plastic bags to clear the volleyball court. (I can hear the collective sneer of men everywhere.)

The job I was in for wasn't elective though. Unless you count the result of a chosen lifestyle. I was getting cut on because things had spread. Bad cells doing bad things.

It's funny. There I was, lying there under the beady lights, waiting for some lab technician with thick glasses and bad breath to come back and tell the doc if things were cool. It's the sins of my youth that had placed me in this predicament, the endless summer days out in the water, surfing, swimming, just plain hanging with my buds on the hot sand. The messenger lab rat had pasty white skin, no wrinkles. Probably served a volleyball under hand. I bet he hadn't been laid in months.

Punk couldn't *earn* the bitch named skin cancer. And I was jealous. This wasn't by-choice surgery. My choice had been to play outside in the sun, all my life, mostly without a hat. Now, *this* was my price, no-free lunch and all that. It wouldn't kill me, but I could end up looking, well … cut and pasted, biophotoshopped.

Somewhere in the take-the-patient's-mind-off-the-procedure conversation, sunscreen entered the dialogue. Oh, you mean that white stuff that the lifeguards put on their nose, like a seagull shit on their beak. Naw. Sunglasses are fine.

We were kids, immortal. We were surfers.

Technically, it wasn't my face under deconstruction, but my nose, which sits on top of the face. I knew that it was commonly felt by most surgeons that a nose is much more difficult to rebuild when sliced and diced away; more difficult than, say, a shoulder or a thigh. With a bad hair style, you can always hide an ear. Noses are tough.

Right down the hall, in the lobby of my next stop after the dermatologist had finished with this "office visit," were half a dozen women thumbing through the pictorials that would shape their future by shaping their flesh. Most of them would be waiting to have the plastic surgeon alter their physical appearance in some way; almost always in an effort to look younger. Nobody goes to a plastic surgeon wanting a more mature look.

I was running from what'd happened in my youth. They were struggling to hold onto theirs.

And as the dermatologist came back in to take "just one more small section" from my left temple ("Let's just snag this little beauty as long as we have you here"), and yet another basal cell carcinoma, ("Oh, nobody dies from these"), the nurse with the soldering gun in tow stood ready, like a gunnery sergeant feeding a string of 50 caliber bullets into a machine gun. She was ready to stop the bleeding by welding the ends of those little bleeders shut.

Why would anyone *choose* to have their body cut into, onto, moving flesh around like clay on a potter's wheel? Why would you make a conscious decision to have someone cut you open? Why not run a few more miles, pad your bra, and put that white crap on your nose? But we know why, I think, the reasons lying inside our subconscious, sandwiched between repressed pain and thrilling anticipation.

The shape of a person's body, especially the face, is the windsock for the rest of their being. We are subtly taught this through our means of socialization, from the school principal's disciplinary scowl, to watching our mothers apply their make up before leaving the house, to the deodorant commercials that feature former *Baywatch* types. A chiseled jaw, man or woman, is external evidence of internal strength and resilience. A furled brow means intensity, worry, sometimes anger. And the eyes, the so-called windows to the soul, they speak volumes that we are unable to hear. If a skilled surgeon can give us what was not a standard feature at birth, tighten up what age, gravity, kids, stress and sun have lowered, then why not, the entitled will ask?

"Raises the self—esteem," we are told, "puts back what should be there." The anecdotes are fast, furious and compelling. I appears that most women who opt for elective surgery state that they need to feel more beautiful for themselves, not those who look at them. More out of compassion for the concept than true understanding, I can almost embrace those claims.

"I love my kids," a woman will say, "but they ruined my boobs."

If I was a woman, listening for 20 years to every other man turn to his friends and say, "Bro, check out that rack," I'd still want to push back and remind men that they make up a high percentage of the Botox market.

Men, face it—it's our own damn fault.

It must be hard to fight that particular stereotype, all that white noise telling women how important mammary glands are. Our society says they should be firm, shapely, and if possible, large. That is *our* society though, an important footnote.

Usually, when a small skin cancer, lesion or mole is removed, the kindly nurses pull down their masks to let you see their sincerity and say it's all fine, the doc will just put a few stitches in the area to keep it shut tight and clean while it heals up and disappears into a small inconvenience of the past.

When the last biopsy report finally came back with "clear margins," I heard none of these benign pleasantries, only, "Well, the plastic surgeon doing the closing is very good." Nurses are healers, they have access to the drift of things to come, whether appealing or appalling.

Dog eat dog, I thought, sun eat skin, skin eat flesh, cut or be killed. No love at all in looking good early, then flaming out.

I tried to comfort myself with the snippet of knowledge that Robert Redford refused to have a face lift against the constant request of movie studio heads.

I knew this was more than a "closing." The removal of the epidermis and dermis layers off my nose had crossed this inconvenience over into the realm of reconstructive surgery, the same type used when someone puts their head through a windshield. Again, my research had told me that noses were the trickiest to get right, whatever that means. You just don't slice off a little piece from your ass or behind your ear and stick in on like play dough. There are things to consider—like blood supply and airways. Aesthetics are nice, but first you have to make sure the flesh and skin you relocate will take to its new location. Ever move a beautiful healthy rose bush to another part of the yard and come back from vacation to find the sucker dead?

In certain indigenous cultures, an elder is given great respect for having earned the deep crevices running down his or her face like vertical rain gutters. Old black and white photos of the great Native American Chiefs show unforgettable features that command respect and knowledge with a knowing sense of grace and compassion. Other tribes around the world will alter their appearance, mostly by piercing and tattoos, to make themselves more desirable to the opposite sex or to display physical prowess.

Walking around college campuses these days, I can't say that the piercing/tattoo thing is much different from Zulu culture or New Hebridean fashion of the 1800's.

The great Apache warrior Geronimo said, "I will fight no more forever."

I promised myself that I would use more sunscreen. Forever.

Interestingly, in the upcoming years disease may finally affect fashion. What some experts are saying is that due to the rapid advancement of skin cancers, within a generation, two at the most, tan skin will no longer be equated with the outdoor leisure class—the athletic types who ski, golf, and ride mountain bikes instead of working real jobs. One has to wonder if at some point our society would return to the pugmarks of a century ago, when pale white skin meant that the individual didn't have to work. They could sit on the veranda all day and sip iced tea. Watching my fifteen-year-old daughter refuse anything higher than sunscreen number seven, I have my reservations.

The cultural ideology of youth-centrism is pervasive, a billion-dollar industry. The myth of immortality has become its own political economy. Kids who've never heard of *The Who* don't necessarily want to die before they get old. But they might consider death before *looking* older.

But what is age anyway? A numerical designation of one human's existence. The tennis icon, Andre Agassi makes the finals of the 2005 U.S. Open at 34 years old. The NY Times labels him, "the geezer of the finals." And arguably, the greatest baseball pitcher of all time, Satchel Paige, who played his last professional game in 1965 at fifty-nine years old, once asked, "How old would you be if you didn't know how old you were?"

I thought I was too young for anything resembling a medical "operation." Too much association with bad stuff. With things that old people need.

Preparing for surgery is an interesting ordeal, sort of a micro version of being inducted into the army. They make sure that you are, in fact, who you say you are, take away your clothes and hand you a generic gown—no different than army fatigues or prison blues. You remove all your jewelry, even the little cross that you had worn around your neck since 6th grade. It's all very humiliating, this deconstruction of one's pride.

And so many forms to sign. Yes, *I* would be the responsible party and pay the bill if my insurance company, whom *I* responsibly paid every month, failed to do so. Yes, *I* would hold harmless all the doctors and nurses who would be working on me. Hey, it's not their fault I was raised a beach rat.

You lie there on the stainless-steel table, lights so bright they seem as if they could worsen your skin cancer just from lying under them. And all sorts of things run through your mind. You are giving up control to a man or a woman who is just like you, but went to school a few more years, men and women who you can't see behind the masks. I would have liked to see a powerfully cut jaw under the sterile garb, not a furled brow behind the glasses. This masked person will decide how you look. The surgeons play God with your flesh. And you breathe the gas that gives them permission.

In the waiting room I had flipped through the generic pamphlets from the American Society of Plastic Surgeons. The one touting forehead lift read, "You'll be very pleased with your refreshed and rejuvenated appearance." Another one on liposuction stated that, "You may notice that clothes fit more comfortably, and you'll feel more confident about your appearance." I wondered if teenagers got much of their confidence from the current trend of baggy clothes. Old men walk my neighborhood and their pants sag in the rear just the same. A cultural bridge, I thought, and wondered if I would mention that to my teenage son.

Oddly, as the minutes ticked away, I was becoming okay with all this. I kept hearing the quote from Dr. Beck Wethers, a member of the ill-fated Everest exhibition where more than a half dozen people died. He had been given up for dead, lost in a blinding snowstorm at 28,000 feet but somehow managed to survive a night outside of the protection of the tents. In the morning, he stumbled, mummy-like, into the morbid camp, most of his extremities already decomposed with frostbite.

Months later, not enough fingers and toes left to count "this-little-piggy" on, he very calmly looked at his interviewer who was wondering, then asking, "What does it feel like?"

It's only body parts, Wethers told him, only body parts.

I knew what had to be done. The plastic surgeon, a likable craftsman with a top-shelf reputation, had shown me a digital picture of my face, sans nose and a good chunk of the left temple; just walked right into the room, opened the file, looked at the photo, showed it to me and said, "Yep, we have some work to do." That honesty was comforting. I like no-bullshit people, especially no-bullshit docs. I could see hanging out with this guy, loaning him tools, trusting his golf score. He seemed the right age: old enough to have some experience but not burnt out on his job.

I signed forms, thought about women getting artificial breasts for Christmas, put on my backless gown, and flashed on kids born with cleft palates. Climbing up onto the operating room table, I suddenly realized how body parts have become action verbs.

"Get a leg up on that project", "Don't try to strong arm him", "Face the music pal; you just have to stomach it", "Have the heart to finger your way through the problem." Beck Wethers' body parts had become part of the vernacular of success, some type of urban legend lexicon.

Suddenly, I was connected to every human being who had been operated on, who had gone under general anesthesia, who had slept the sleep of the chemically induced necessity.

I was egoless because I had no choice. Forced Zen was better than none at all.

And at that moment I realized that wounds resonate in some shared experience. That violation of external integrity creates an internal bond for all those who are affected. But they must accept it. If I was to look like the elephant man, I would need some training.

I was reminded of a friend who died twice so that he could live once—the first time when hit by a bus resulting in the loss of a leg, and again when he was struck by a truck causing his paralysis from the chest down.

"Oedipus," he would always say, "was haunted by a wound for which he had no basis of fear. And a denial of one's wound is like a denial of one's life." Where does strength like this come from? The body is only a carrier he would tell me in moments of quiet reflection. What was I carrying around inside me that needing anything but a hole in my face that let air in and air out? The importance of shape began to lose its import.

A precise moment finds a precise feeling. But the whole paradigm was still a bit cloudy. In my internal struggle I was hoping for a precision job, while losing my disdain for elective surgery, remembering all the while that the surgeon had told me, "The cosmetic funds the reconstructive."

Hey, people are lucky to have choices. They want liposuction. Fine. Go for it. If I opt to run 60 miles a week, eat less and look at silicone boobs in a whole new light, well, that's not hard either.

Yes sir, the choices are good.

Something heroic collided with a real-life reality TV show. Against all odds, maybe I was growing up—maturity moving in like a metaphor. The far-reaching fun, the sun, the sins, the unparalleled joy tailored behind me, in sync. Just so long as I didn't make any sudden moves under the knife.

This augmentation of my own had given me this unique relationship with any man or woman who electively chooses a change in their appearance. It would connect me to every cosmetic surgery ever performed, no matter the reason or rationale behind it. I gained more empathy for my female friends who opted for breast augmentation. They looked better in a swimsuit but more importantly, they felt better about themselves generally.

Our complimentary wounds did not come at the hand of fate behind the bumper of a truck; they were lifestyle-catalyzed, one backward, one forward.

I asked my surgeon if he would rather stick to the more altruistic side of his chosen profession, just focusing on the necessary things like mugs torn up in car crashes and noses lost to the Endless Summer.

"Sure," he replied, "but then I'd be driving an old car like yours."

And who was I to judge? My wife, who chose to breast feed our two kids, perhaps lost some of the shapeliness of her amazing figure in service of the right decision for our offspring. Her body, her choice. She will likely never opt for silicone; it's not in her nature. But as one of my friends once suggested in jest, "I could probably come to like a pair of those firm, perky bolt-ons, but the novelty would wear off like a new pair of sunglasses that scratch."

The locker-room crassness bothered me but I could sense the overt heterogeneity that's been ingrained in our culture.

There are those who say that the human body is only a vehicle for the soul. You can believe that or not. But there is no denying that it will decompose at some point. The Egyptians worked really hard to slow that process. And the Indiana Jones types had a field day peeling off the layers. Still, those people had indeed checked out a long time ago, with or without souls.

Like everybody, I don't want to live out my sunset years battling some chronic disease. I don't smoke, eat healthily, drink only in moderation, and exercise more than regularly. The stress is kept in check and other than a few aches and pains (and surgeries) from time to time, I seem to be moving through the mid-way mark better than most.

Okay, the sun is turning my face into the cracked dashboard of a '67 Buick Skylark left in a Phoenix backyard. But with a bag over my head or a 10k race to run, I can pass for half my age. Considering my active past, I would rather be run over by a Marlboro truck, that large picture of a rugged cowboy staring down on me from the side flashing my last view on earth, than struggling with the Big C or chronic pulmonary disease for the last five or ten years of life. It's not so much the fear of pain, but more the inconvenience of it all. I would feel like I failed, like I should have gone out the way I lived, in a fiery ball; better too. As Neil Young said, "To *burn out than fade away.*"

Physical reification is not a course taught in grad school, and we cannot touch the brakes of our lives the same way we touch the dreams in our heads.

I told the doc I just wanted local anesthesia. He laughed and said no I didn't. How about a halfway thing, like they do when they pull out wisdom teeth? That would be my choice, but he would be doing some intricate work around my face—ship-in-a-bottle stuff. If I became irritable, itchy, and squirmy or pissed off, I could screw up his concentration and then they'd knock me out anyway.

"Shit," I thought, "then knock my ass out. But I'm not staying overnight. And when can I get back into the water? There was a good south swell due to hit."

"Talk to me Beck Wethers. Hey doc, measure twice, cut once."

"Kid," he said, "You cannot be simultaneously dispassionate, dry, emotionless, imperturbable, indifferent, indurated, unexcitable, passionless, phlegmatic, placid, poker-faced, reserved, reticent, self-contained, stoic, stolid, taciturn, unconcerned, unemotional, unexcitable, unfeeling, unflappable and god damn concerned about how your frickin' face will look after I pour my heart and twenty years of skill into it." And as I looked up into the cool, steely blue eyes of the anesthesiologist, I nodded, said he was slowly melding conversation with conversion and counted backwards from 10 to 9 to 8 to …

When I woke up in post op, I felt as if I had been on a three-day tequila bender in Tijuana—bent, spun, oozing from newfound holes in my body, bleeding pale memories of where I was, who I had been with? Did I choose this? Earn it? Or deserve it? Trying to talk, the words slithering out of my mouth at a fresh-faced nurse, no mask covering her kind words … well?

"It went great. You'll be happy." Cool. Chicks dig … oh, never mind. Where's my shorts and T-shirt? No offense, but I'd kindly like to get the fuck out of here. This place makes me nervous.

I have a nose again, and a degree of bilateral appearance between the sides of my temples. They're not pretty, but I never was. I won't be doing underwear commercials, but the nose works. Air goes in, air comes out. Even that Marlboro Man is air-brushed rugged on purpose.

And my wounds make me unique and connected.

James Hillman (Suicide and the Soul, 1965) suggests to us that the place where we are most vulnerable must be most venerated, "for they mark a sacred place in us that we would have ignored."

A broken heart over a failed love affair comes to mind. But so does that white shit that lifeguards wear on their nose.

The flesh moved deftly by my new-best-friend, the surgeon, from one side of my nose to the tip, seems to be holding up so far. The scars will improve with time, fading to a feint reminder of some false sense of youthful immortality. More skin cancers will appear, and I will deal with them as I must. Sadly, hundreds of thousands are walking around in the same position.

My enlightened friend in a wheelchair says I look like an Irish alcoholic that was in a bar room knife fight——an image that is not too far from where I could've ended up. I just got there early.

And artificially.

I realized that Kant was right. If I am but a member of humanity, no perfectly straight thing will ever be made of this crooked, sun-burnt timber.

I've made my peace with silicone.

Prescript: This essay first appeared in my book, Finding Triathlon (Hatherleigh, 2015). I'd forgotten I wrote it until a colleague who knew of my recent open-heart surgery sent it to me. The protagonist, Big Jim, is gone now. But my rebuilt heart is doing well, and the sprinklers keep things green and lush. I think of Jim now and then; the way he sauntered down the block in the pre-dawn chill wearing only a t-shirt and shorts. And in the heat of summer, working shirtless in his yard, that reddish, ropey, train-track scar running down his chest. I'd like to trade cardiac rehab stories with Big Jim not because I think he's smart or caring. More so because he earned the conversation. I suppose a big part of a good rehab is finding others who have been where you are right now, who've suffered from injury, illness, lost limbs, lost love, lost homes, lost jobs … who have earned the conversation. Say all you want about the awkward group-circles found in everything from AA meetings to ZZ Top fan gatherings. Truth is, I couldn't imagine going through rehab from ANYTHING without the benefit of others who've lost, loved, struggled, and survived.

The Heart of the Matter

You can spend great periods of time thinking about sport and in particular just what makes an endurance athlete. It happens to me a lot.

The last time was in late December, and the sun was low and cold, and my thoughts were casting long shadows. It was my neighbor, Big Jim; he was the one who'd brought it on by challenging me to identify a single illuminating principle of endurance sports; one idea around which he could suspend his disbelief.

"C'mon, Tinley" he goaded, "I used to see you and your pals running in the rain and riding across eight zip codes while I pushed paper across my desk. Just give this sedentary soul one generalized concept of why you endurance freaks do what you do."

It was a valid if not heartfelt prompt and hard as tried I couldn't conjure a worthy reply nor offer something without skirting into some mediated phrase as "well, it depends."

One thing, one reason, one central idea ... that's all Big Jim asked as I stood in the front yard and had no singular pathway to the heart of the matter. Stumped, scanning the shadows as they crept eastward, I wanted an easy out, a plea bargain based on something ethereal and flaky. It was getting cold, and I wanted to go inside. But Big Jim had helped me fix my sprinklers that day and I shrugged and mumbled something weak and watery about us *just following our hearts* before turning toward the door. Jim tactfully parried with a quote from Lincoln: "He has the right to criticize who has the heart to help."

Big Jim's heart had my thirsty plants bowing in praise. We owed him something.

In recognition of the three hours his hands had dug in my yard, I faced him full up and said I was going to think about it. Then his sweetheart-of-a-wife walked by and pulled two Mexican beers out of a sack like a magician finds a coin beyond your ear. This is why people don't move, I thought. It has nothing to do with job changes or downsizing a house. You stay in the same neighborhood for 25 years for the magical Mexican beer trick.

"Now, Big Jim, it's like this" ... and I started in with my feigned Intro to Physiology lesson about cardiac stroke volume and ATP production and oxygen uptake and catecholamine release, all of which caused him to do what any man does when he loses interest in a conversation—he peels the label off the beer bottle.

Right then Big Jim sat down on the curb, a sure sign that he wasn't happy with me trying to substitute mechanics for motive. "Look, hotshot" his right eye held my two while he studied the gold and brown label with the other. "What's the most flattering thing you can say about another athlete?"

"Ah, that's easy," I sipped from my Bohemia and took his toss. "Any athlete will say the same—*he's got heart*—that's the biggest compliment a peer can offer."

Big Jim stood, pulling up his sagging Wranglers and wiping his hands behind the knees. He said he was going home for supper and thanks for making it perfectly clear why people ran and swam and biked and skied across deserts for "reasons only reason understands."

And then he limped away, mumbling Homer Simpson-like, "hmmm, heart of the matter."

He'd known all along, of course. It was a brilliant tactic from a man who has trouble walking to the end of the block. And he knew that I knew it but couldn't quite remember it. Because when talking about anything from the moment of conception to the end of earthly life, the heart—from all points of science, study and approach to knowledge—is a central point of departure, regardless of which direction that you are headed. And no less can be said about its role in endurance sports.

If broken from a failed relationship, we can still run miles and miles in an effort to heal it. If we soar from some grand victory, we can still feel it break when others who live inside our own cannot share that glee. If we wear it on our sleeves, we must be ready to take that which others can sling at us. And if we keep it too closely guarded, we rarely reach the peaks and valleys of human emotion.

The four chambers of the heart drive the fluid that delivers the goods to the muscles that make us go. Blood moves as a clock to the points of the bodily compass. Kids understand this. Adults suffer the consequences of forgetting it. The heart can gush with pleasure if all systems move in sync or stop us cold in our tracks if dammed by the particulars of age and treason of poor choice.

The heart can be observed, dissected, broken, repaired and replaced. We rely on it like a good neighbor, realizing that even if it's always there doing what it's supposed to, we still need to pay attention to it.

To succeed in endurance sport and in life all you need is a big heart that has nothing to do with size.

When I saw Big Jim in the morning, he was out front admiring our sprinkler repair.

"We might need to replace that valve up near the big tree before too long."

I asked him if he wanted to walk to the end of the block.

Prescript: Sometimes rehab doesn't work; it doesn't save the affected from injury, illness, excess or their own internal demons. Shortly after the actor and comedian Robin Williams committed suicide on August 11th, 2014, I was tasked with making sense of senselessness. Robin and I had become friends who shared a love of cycling. He'd spoken privately and publicly of his challenges with drugs and alcohol, going so far as to claim, "I went to rehab in the wine country. You know, just to keep my options open." One can only guess why his times in formal rehabilitation were unable to move his mind far enough away from his fateful choice. Robin's story is a sobering reminder that at best, rehabilitation in any form is simply an effort to improve. To go on living as best we can, given our challenges.

Channeling Pain, Pleasure, and the People: The Tormented Gift of Robin Williams

"I think now, looking back, we did not fight the enemy; we fought ourselves. And the enemy was in us.

—From Chris Taylor (Charlie Sheen) in Platoon (1986)

The Treason of the Artist

In Arthurian legend, the *Fisher King* is one of a long line of protectors of the Holy Grail. But this King is wounded, emasculated in such a disguised fashion that he continues to protect the Grail but cannot father an heir in his impotence. His weakness, visibly affecting the health and strength of his kingdom, causes him much suffering. But still, he protects the Grail, waits for someone to heal him, and fishes at the river.

For Robin Williams, the actor-comedic who opted out of life on 8/11/14, a vital and viral artistic king, depression was his impotence. His ultimate choice exposed how the protector role, once again, does nothing unless deeper root problems are exposed. And addressed.

Pundits have offered thoughts on the intersections of Williams' acting and comedic skills, his mental state, and his profound body of work—over eighty films in three decades. The demons that visited his head, some have voyeuristically argued, are the catalysts that generated his genius. And while there is little doubt that his amazing wit and intellect, when applied to popular culture references and offered through his intricate impressions … these were the foundations of that manic style of rapid-fire comedy.

But, for this friend and fan, it was his dramatic roles that showed humanity and the spirit of his life. This is where his inner battles were waged for the world to see. These roles—when the perfect pain comes in contact with the perfect part—are the treason of the artist: Jim Morrison singing *The End*, Picasso's *Starry, Starry Night*, Frida Kahlo's *The Two Fridas*, Lou Gehrig's *Luckiest Man in the World speech*, Roosevelt's *A day that will live in infamy* claim, and David Foster Wallace's *Infinite Jest*. So, when Robin Williams tells Matt Damon's character in the film *Good Will Hunting* that, "*You're a genius, Will. No one denies that. No one could possibly understand the depths of you,*" we might ask who Williams is speaking to or about.

As fans, we fail to see the pain hiding just behind the devouring eye; we fail to see the associated torment of artistic brilliance. And the artist is always on stage, offering things they must. For they are always and already on the cusp of madness. We just never see it.

Ursula K. Le Guin argues in her seminal work, *Those Who Walk Away from Omelas*, that "only pain is intellectual, only evil interesting." For the artist trading pointy edges with the pain of addiction, depression, and *is-it-all-worth-it* questions, these roles act as a kind of release valve for their suffering. And in some odd marriage of production and consumption, the fan consumes the metaphor for their own disparate but connected lives. Thus, Hemingway's foray into the vagaries of the Spanish War function on the same level as Kurt Cobain's lyrics from his song, *Downer*:

> *Butchered sincerity, act out of loyalty*
> *Defend your true country, wish away pain*
> *Hand out lobotomies, to save little families*
> *Surrealistic fantasy, bland, boring, pain.*

The artist's work is a test for what might be a normal life. But the paradox returns when the fan responds with "they were just brilliant in that role." Were they acting, we might ask, or projecting a need to find some essential normalcy?

Eugene O'Neill's *The Iceman Cometh*, Charlie Parker's *Ornithology*, Robin Williams in *The Fisher King* wondering why we haven't learned the musical lessons of John Lennon to give peace a chance—these are the brilliance of our artistic composers. But hidden in those performances—whether real or imagined—is what Le Guin calls "the banality of evil, and the terrible boredom of pain." That is the treason few see and fewer feel, buried beneath the rubble of material wealth and immaterial fame.

And so, when the spot-lit star enters "rehab" we are left knowing nothing other than they must not have been able to heal themselves without professional support. And we root for their success and return if only to show the Everyman that these geniuses are as failingly human as the rest of us.

To Be King, Just for a Day

Few of us fully understand the perils of a vaulted existence. Many of the fallen artistic heroes have surrendered wholly to the pursuit of earthly greatness, exposing them to the terrifying process of public ruination when failed morality and the ravages of physical decline or extinguish come to collect. They suffer both in their boot-strapped quests and their ignominious return to regularity. All for the chance to be king. And most say they wouldn't change a thing. When they fail as royalty, they are laid bare on the altar of social media. And suddenly they have ten thousand new best friends who could have saved them.

(Insert celebrity here) died and the carrion swoop. Copters, cameras, and commercial talking heads stabbing and dodging; the natural commoditization of an (un)natural death sets in motion the fallen hero machine. Life becomes as thin as the green paper that drives the Industrial Celebrity Complex. Think Kobe. Think Marilyn Monroe. Consider that JFK's death has become its own industry.

And "ah, geez," the populace suggest. "If only he would've called me. I could've taken him out for a few beers and eased his pain. I'm not famous but hell ... I've been down."

I never drank with Robin Williams. But I drank for him.

==

The story of Robin Williams is the story of a man both conflicted and divided; that tormented genius who sought anonymity on a bike or a treadmill or a walk in the woods. Who only wanted to be *one-of-the-guys.* On one of our first bike rides together, we stopped for coffee and some yahoo asked for the Scottish Golf Skit. "*Give it to us, Robin!*" The barrister rolled her eyes and flashed Robin a few Tiburon, CA gang signs.

"It's okay," her fingers signaled, "He's just another 27-year-old wonder-geek who sold his start-up app for eight figures."

On the way home, held up at a red light, a dark-haired beauty hailed from a minivan, "luv you long time, Robin," and pulled her tube top down past her ponytail as the light changed to green and the kids drooled from the 2nd and 3rd row seats.

"Is this the way it works, Robin?" I asked." You're on stage 24/7?"

"Every day. Every. Fucking. Hour."

"Is it worth it?"

"Can't see that I have a choice. And I'm good. You know? And I love it. Did I say that I'm good?"

"It's good to be king, eh Capitan oh my slow riding Captain."

"Fuck off, Tinley."

An essential difference in leadership, regardless of the platform or effect, is in motive. Some kings are effective for their results however managed and attained. Others are successful because they do it for the right reasons. Robin Williams was successful in his roles because they weren't roles. Just extensions of his being. Using not just his fame but the strategy of being famous, Williams effected positive change in many of those who struggled with more obvious bad hands dealt. I sometimes wonder if Robin's rehab failed because they required just too much veracity as if his counselors wouldn't allow his release valve that was his role playing. Still, his legacy of roles is un-mutable.

In a darkened hospital room, here's Robin holding the flesh-eaten stumps of a young woman as if they were beautifully manicured hands while the nurses want to hear him do Mork's nano-nano one more time. Here's Robin defending Lance Armstrong not because he wants to offer an opinion on Armstrong's use of performance enhancing drugs but because he sees Lance as a survivor, as a kid from a fucked-up home who beat the cancer bitch. Here's Robin bleeding empathy for the physically challenged and the cancer- ridden, and the homeless, and the socially beat-to-shit not because they looked like him but because beneath that entire comedic front, there was still the pain. And it was his to negotiate.

In many ways, Robin's foray into altruism, his platformed-use to make a difference, to heal those in need ... to me, that was his ongoing attempt to find relief from his own anguish and need.

Suicide and the Hardest Town Played

The country singer, Tom T. Hall, writes about this tenderfoot communion between artists and their followers in his insightful song, *Last Hard Town*. "They came to see the people that they thought we were and never changed their minds," adding the admission that "what a picker does for others is the thing he's mainly doing for himself" (Hall, 1973). For Robin Williams, his connection to the Everyman, the under-represented, the physically challenged, and the fallen hero, suggests a response to Hall's argument that no one really knows the celebrity. The fans only know what they want to know.

But watch this boys and girls: Here's the Funny Man marching through cancer wards late at night with nary a camera or PR prop insight. Here's Williams being more than human because this is the best way he knows how to battle the bad hand of depression that he has been dealt. Williams' altruism, while perfectly authentic, just might've carried the additional burden as some disguised plea for help.

Hey folks, I'm doing this because I do care. But I'm also channeling their pain on top of my own. Can't anyone see it? I am the Wounded King who has been tasked with protecting and entertaining those who can't protect and amuse themselves. Does anyone else want this job? Because I just don't know how long I can carry the burden.

And for those who have never felt what David Foster Wallace called "the invisible agony," that ten-ton darkness pressing in from all points, this writer pleads compassion for depression, compassion for suicide, and compassion for Robin's choice.

As Wallace, who made his own suicidal choice on September 12, 2008, suggests, "Make no mistake about people who leap from burning windows. Their terror of falling from a great height is still just as great as it would be for you or me standing speculatively at the same window just checking out the view; the fear of falling remains a constant. The variable here is the other terror, the fire's flames: when the flames get close enough, falling to death becomes the slightly less terrible of two terrors."

If living with depression was the more terrible of Robin Williams' options then I suggest in both respect and humanness, we celebrate the near limitless pleasure he brought millions and find ways of addressing that invisible agony he faced. We celebrate the effects of how he fought the good fight. Because in the wake of those tormented battles came his humanity which is a humanity that is missed. And much needed.

Williams might've thought his race was run, his journey bereft of moral completion. He was no longer vital; his depressed voice might've suggested. His TV series was canceled. Kids through college. Occupational pugmarks checked on the way to banality. But what Robin missed is what most of us miss in our search for redemption. It's what he acted in *The Fisher King*. Our acceptance of our own fallacies, our own depressions, our own humanness, our own living legacy.

There is one image I have of our times together, of Robin leaning into the pre-teen, physically challenged lad, Rudy Garcia-Tolson, a boy born without some parts of lower legs who chose to have the rest simply discarded because, as he would suggest, they just got in the way. Williams looks around the glitterati and the beautiful able-bodied collective at some high-end sporting ceremony and tells the young Garcia-Tolson that it is he, a soulful kid who is more whole than the posturing and pretension abounding.

"Money and legs," I think he said, "are over-rated, Rudy. Keep your soul instead."

I don't know what Robin forgot to keep. I just miss my friend.

"The war is over for me now, but it will always be there … for what Rhah called possession of my soul. There are times since I've felt like the child born of those two fathers. But be that as it may, those of us who did make it have an obligation to build again, to teach to others what we know, and to try with what's left of our lives to find goodness and a meaning to this life."

—From Chris Taylor (Charlie Sheen) in Platoon (1986)

Playing Through

I first saw Jeremey Poincinot on the back of a tandem bike. It was an organized ride by Challenged Athletes Foundation; maybe 50 or 60 of us on a three-day spin through Northern California's wine country. I rode up next to the tandem and said something inane like "nothing like a friend" or "two for the price of one." I'm sure it was cheesy with a hidden note of sarcasm. Jeremey, sitting in the back, looked my way and asked, "Who's that?" That evening he was the guest speaker at dinner and halfway through his talk, I turned to my wife and said, "I wanna hang out with that guy."

I came to learn that Jeremey had lost his sight while a 19-year-old student at San Diego State University. After months of misdiagnosis, it was determined that he had Leber's hereditary optic neuropathy, a rare inherited pathology that effects mostly teen males. Jeremey lost most of his central vision and was pronounced legally blind. Unable to drive or recognize people in an instance, his life was forever changed.

Though he had excelled at golf before the disease, Jeremey at first resisted a return to golf or any sport. But upon the encouragement of his parents, Poincinot found and excelled at blind golf, eventually winning three world championships in his category. He now works as a successful inspirational speaker, traveling the world, telling his tale of resiliency and courage. One of the first times I invited him to speak at SDSU, the university where he eventually graduated from and where I have been teaching for nearly two decades, on the way back from his talk to my car, he suggested we stop into his old fraternity house. For some reason this made me nervous:

Jeremey: Hey, do you mind if we swing by the frat house for a minute?

Translation: We'll be there for several hours.

Me: Don't you want to get home and see your family?

Translation: I want to get home and see my family.

Jeremey: I'm sure no one will remember me.

Translation: I will be a rock star.

Me: Alright, but if they offer us a drink we should decline.

Translation: I hope they offer us something to drink.

Jeremey: We all outgrow our college years at some point.

Translation: We are frat brothers for life.

We ended up having a good time and I got to see the inside of a fraternity house for the first time in 40 years. The residents were cordial, bordering on gushing to Jeremey and a bit fearful of a professor in their digs. The following is my conversation with Jeremey.

ST: What was your first reaction when you were told that your sight wasn't going to improve?

JP: So, there were multiple months, like two to three months, where I lived in a purgatory, where I thought that I was gonna see again because doctors didn't know what it was. So, I was misdiagnosed with several things. So, I had a spinal tap done. And the doctor said, "You have a classic case of something called optic neuritis, which is inflammation of the optic nerves. So, we're gonna pump steroids into you every day for five days, and that'll minimize the inflammation. You'll be fine." I was telling my fraternity brothers like, five years from now we're gonna laugh at this because I'll be able to see. And then it didn't work out that way. Then the docs thought I had something called NMO. So, I got the treatment for that. Well, then they said I was gonna become paraplegic and go blind with that. But the treatment for that was a catheter in my jugular and they did something called plasma pheresis. So, I did all these things expecting to see again. But there was no real definitive diagnosis until they identified that it was LHON, Leber's Hereditary Optic Neuropathy.

ST: How do you feel now, reflecting on that diagnosis that had no known cure? Do you think that at least knowing what you were up against had any bearing on your rehabilitation?

JP: I think it was like, okay; now we know. It's at least nice to have a diagnosis and know what the heck's going on. But yeah, there's here's a little bit of honesty. At that point I just kind of ... I didn't care. I didn't care anymore. I didn't care about life. I didn't. Nothing felt real. I felt like I was just living a long nightmare. And I was hoping I would one day see again, or wake up from it and see and go, "Wow! That was such a trip." But yeah, it was weird. When I got the diagnosis, it was ... it was nice to get a diagnosis, but it was also like this all isn't real, and this kind of just sucks and to add insult to injury, I don't really care anymore. I was very apathetic at that point about life.

ST: What was that period of adjustment like; those early weeks and months of your rehab? Could you gradually wrap your head around your future? Or were you still reeling from all the failed tests that were used to determine a correct diagnosis?

JP: It's hard to say. I don't wish it on people ever. The spinal tap was whatever. But the catheter in my hand for five days was annoying. And the one in my jugular for 10 days was even worse. I would have been okay. I think I would have been just fine had I not gone through those things. I don't know if you know, but my sister lost her sight five years ago. But she didn't have to go through all those misdiagnoses. And I feel like, yeah, I'd rather have not gone through those things. Still, it's a rapid onset of blindness. I went legally blind in two or three months, and it shouldn't get worse. So at least if you said, "Hey kid, you're legally blind," It was hard hitting and fast. I feel like it would be harder if it was a progressive sight loss journey where, "Hey, in 10 years you're gonna become totally blind." I couldn't imagine that. Going through those experiences honestly, just made me more and more numb to what the hell was going on. It was just like; I don't even care anymore. Like you can just tell me I have whatever. I just don't even care. I was numb and apathetic, and just had no zest in my being anymore. It was just like it was all taken from me.

ST. Was there a moment or a week when you realized that you could remain in this vacuous period, this numbness you talk about forever? Or was there, uh, what's that line from the film Shawshank Redemption? Get busy living or get busy dying.

JP: Yeah, I think there was. It was an accumulation of things. But if I was gonna put it on one pivotal moment. It was the story I talk about in presentations where the F 18 plane crash landed in San Diego, and four people died. And it was a man's wife, his mother-in-law, and of his two children that died. That kind of that shook me and provided immediate perspective and made me go "Whoa! That guy lost four family members. And I'm just legally blind." I just started to say to myself things could be worse. And then that was my new mantra. I started to live like things could be worse. Does it suck? Absolutely. But things could be worse. I needed to realize that. That was one of the most pivotal things for me. All right, you gotta kind of buck up, kid, because this, this is not the end of the world.

ST: Yeah, I think they call that "catastrophizing" or at least that's one term for it. And it seems to be a common theme amongst people who, when they're going through rehabilitation, they use that strategy you just spoke of. They start to think, "Gosh! You know it really could be a lot worse. So, even though I'm bad off, I still have a lot to live for."

JP: Right. And I sort of think, man, like as long as you're above ground, as long as you're living, things could be worse. I just couldn't imagine what that guy who lost his family went through. It's not so insurmountable, but it's one of those things where you think, would you rather go legally blind than lose four family members? And it's horrible to think that way, but it definitely puts things into perspective to make you go. "Whoa! I gotta stop complaining like, it's not the end of the world. I'm gonna be alright. I gotta find a way to get through this."

ST: How did you feel about your support system at the time? Your family, your friends … the people that you talk about on a regular basis? Could you imagine getting through your issues without them?

JP: No chance. Well, not no chance, but like no way it would have been the same. My rehab wouldn't have happened as soon as it did, and I wouldn't have said I accepted and adjusted and adapted to this until, like at least a year, maybe a year and a half to where I was like "Alright like it is what it is now." But there's no way it would have happened that quickly had I not had the support I had from my family and my friends. It's like in the moment you don't fully understand it. I don't think you're as grateful for it as you should be. But it's easy to look back. It's easier to look back on it and go. My parents were great, my siblings were great, my friends were great, but in that moment, again, I was numb and apathetic, and I wasn't as appreciative. It's hard to be appreciative of the support when you're so bummed out about what is taking place.

ST: I totally get that part, just having my sister and my wife and my kids in the ICU for 5 days. And I'm just saying, I'm okay. I'm okay. You guys don't have to be here. But then they leave, and I'm kinda like staring at the ceiling, going well, now there's no one to talk to.

JP: Yeah, yeah, yeah. And it's like, you know, someone came to me and goes "Wow, how supportive your parents and your siblings and your friends are. How cool is that?" And I go "Yeah, but I'm blind and I'm sorry." I have a hard time appreciating how cool that is when I was just so caught up in what's happened to me. I don't know if that's selfish, but it's just like I'm so bummed out about going legally blind that I have a hard time appreciating the good stuff.

ST: I think they call that being human. Did you ever identify any personal traits you have that enabled you and made your return easier? Just part of your basic personality, or things that you've learned along the way that if you hadn't had that skill, your rehab would've been tougher?

JP: Yeah, I think two things. I think I'm innately optimistic. And I think I'm innately resilient. I'm optimistic, like, I've always been a glass half full kind of guy; let's try to see the positives and things. Because I mean, come on, we're only living once. What's the point in being pessimistic? What's the point in complaining? What's the point in finding the negatives when it's on us to choose how we see things unintended. And I choose to see things from a better perspective. Honestly, I think, being a golfer you kind of build resilience a little bit because it's not a game of perfection. You're gonna make double bogeys. You're gonna have bad shots and it's kind of ... you gotta just keep going and plugging along. And you know, losing my sight was like a quadruple quintuple bogey. But I gotta play the next hole and the next hole and the next hole, and you gotta find a way to be resilient. And so, I think I'm a resilient optimist, and I think those were things that have really helped me get to where I am.

ST: And probably has continued to help you in your occupation and your life. Whether it's family, health, etc., going forward. Think about all the people that fall off the wagon, so to speak. You must have had moments where you felt like it was a setback, a double bogey. You think, "Oh, I'm gonna get involved here. I'm gonna do this. I'm gonna do that." And then in the cold, harsh dawn you realize, "Guess what? I'm still fucking blind." You can have all this resiliency and this positiveness but oops … maybe that's not enough.

JP: Oh, yeah, 100 percent, like I was starting to feel okay. I was stacking up good days like I would have one good day in a week, and I was like stoked about it. And then I'd have two good days in a week, and I was stoked. And then the next week I only have one good day. I was just trying to stack good days, and I remember a time in college when two of my fraternity brothers and said, "Hey, let's go drive up to Laguna Beach for two days, and we're gonna go spend the day up there and go spend the night and just hang and get out of this San Diego State bubble we were in." We were going to go on a Wednesday, but this was Monday when we decided it, and I didn't have much to look forward to during that time. That's all I was excited about. And so Monday I was stoked about it. Tuesday I was stoked about it. And then, like Tuesday evening, one of my buddies was like, "Hey, I got a big test I got to study for. So, I actually can't do it anymore." And that crushed me because I can't drive. I can't say all good dude. I'll still go by myself, or you know it was just a quick reality check to make me realize, like, yeah, I'm still blind, and I can't do some of the things that I used to be able to do. So, yeah I had setbacks like that. I had, you know, people make comments or experiences not go the way I would've like. People might assume or call me out, or think that I was lying to them, that when I told them I was legally blind they'd tell me I was I was lying to them. And that's just extremely uncomfortable, because it's like I'm kind of getting vulnerable here with you and telling you that I'm legally blind, and for you to come back and say no, you're not, you're lying to me.

ST: But blindness as a pathology is much different than missing an arm or leg or being deformed. Or you're going through cancer where your whole body is ravaged, and the outward physical appearance is radically different. You probably don't look any different without your sight.

JP: I have an invisible disability. Which makes it harder because the onus is on me to tell you I can't see it, and I don't always want to tell you. But then, when I do tell somebody there is a connection. The best way for someone to respond is, "Oh, thank you so much for telling me. Is there anything I can do to support you." That's the best way someone can respond. But then you have people who choose the worst way. They claim, "No, you're not." That's the worst way you can respond, and I've had more than I'd like to admit. But then you have people who think they have good intentions. They think they're being supportive, but they'll just grab my arm and start to pull me, and I go, "Whoa! Like I'm not totally blind, and you pulling me is not the best way to support me. Would you want me to just grab you and pull you?" But people think that's the best way. I tell people I'm legally blind and I've had a hundred different responses to it.

ST: I've got a neighbor that I ride my bike with, and he knows about my own vision challenge; he knows that I'm legally blind in my left eye. And so, he always rides on my left, and no matter where we go, he just finds a way to be on my left. Never says anything, never asks, is just always on my left.

JP: What an empathetic human being to be that courteous and thoughtful to think like that. I have those handful of friends that will do things like that and not say anything about it. And they're just stepping up in ways that really do make a difference.

ST: There's a single leg amputee named Paul Martin. I don't know whether you've ever crossed paths with him. He was involved with Challenged Athletes Foundation in the early days. He lost his lower limb in a motorcycle accident. He wrote this book called One Man's Leg, and in it he argued that his life is much better, more interesting being a single leg amputee. I know that some people who have faced these kinds of major challenges say the same thing. Other people say, no, no, that's just rhetoric, that's just them, you know, being inspirational, saying something for the crowd and in their heart of hearts, they wish to be normal. How do you feel about that?

JP: Yeah, it's a good question and I say that in my talks, if you were to offer me my sight back, I wouldn't take it. And I do mean it. I do. I think my life is a lot more interesting being legally blind than it was when I was sighted. In a world full of vanilla, it's kind of nice to not be vanilla. It's nice to be a little different. I definitely see things from a different perspective. Pun intended. But I think there's a fine line where I would like my sight back today. But would I want to go back in time and relive the experience? No, I feel like I've run the marathon across the finish line. Got the metal and the T-shirt. And like, I said, adapted. So, it's my new normal.

I'm comfortable with it. It's a part of my identity. I'm Jeremy Poincinot. I'm legally blind and it is what it is. It's fine. I have no fear behind that anymore. So yeah, like, I wouldn't take my sight back.

ST: That makes perfect sense. I had a retinal specialist tell me that there are optic pathologies where people get back some or all of the sight they've lost after months, weeks, and sometimes even years. And those people claim that once they've adapted to being challenged with their sight and now, I have to adjust again … they complain. Personally, I'd kill for even 2/40 vision in my bad eye.

JP: The only thing I really would want to do is drive. I'd enjoy the ability to drive. Driving is such a necessity in America, and especially in the suburbs. That's the one thing I wish I could do. I would love to be able to have independence and the ability to just drive and go where I want when I want. There's nothing else that I want. The only other thing is with, like my kiddos is to see them playing sports a little better. I'm not gonna be able to play catch with my sons. They can roll me grounders, and then I can throw them balls. But like that's not gonna help them when they're throwing. So, we'll do it in different ways, like I'll make them throw the ball at a mattress. And then I'll catch it when it bounces. I'll get it off the mattress and then throw it back to them.

ST: You talked a little bit about having been a skilled golfer before, and what that might have taught you with respect to resiliency. Can you imagine if you hadn't had golf before and hadn't found and excelled at blind golf? Would you have found something else or was that just the stars all lining up?

JP: If I didn't find blind golf, I would have hoped to have found something because yeah, blind golf gave me something to look forward to during a time I wasn't looking forward to anything. And to be honest, the first time I learned about blind golf, I thought it was a joke. I didn't want to do it. I was anti the idea of it, because I had an expectation level of how I could play golf when I was sighted. I knew that when I lost my sight, I wasn't going to be anywhere near as good, so I kind of didn't want to embarrass myself. And so, I was kind of against the idea of it at first. But after a period of time, and I digested it and let it sink in, I was like, "Alright, I'll give it a shot" and I did, and was like, "Alright. This wasn't as bad as I thought." And then it's kind of become what it is today. It's a little part of my identity; it's something I'm so passionate about, obsessed with and love. I would say, golf sped up my recovery process because it gave me something to look forward to. It gave me something to work on. It gave me something to think about other than my site loss. Because when I lost my site, that's all I thought about.

ST: I was thinking about everyone's rehab and how we want to remember all the positives, all the struggles. But not all the pain. When in rehabilitation, we might repress parts of our struggles into some deep, dark cavern of the mind. But then on occasion, use the wisdom learned at some point; roll that darkness into the light. Do you ever channel your repressed pain into your motivational talks?

JP: Yes, for sure. I tell people about what I went through without boring them to death. And they relate to their own struggles and what was either a good thing for them or what hurt a lot, and what part of their entire healing process is worth remembering. But now it's like, how cool is it I get paid to be a speaker?

ST: If you had to compare your loss of sight to any of your other life challenges or the challenges of people close to you, or even things you've heard about or read about, what similarities have you noticed?

JP: I don't know if I have a good answer. The thing that comes to mind is just having an invisible disability. You have to share the story. The onus is on me to make my tale relevant. That's what I tell other folks who are legally blind "Hey, the onus is on us to disclose it and share it, and I know it can be an uncomfortable thing." For example, you're not gonna preboard on a Southwest flight if you don't tell them you're legally blind. You're not gonna get the accommodation you need or want if you don't advocate for yourself. Because we don't have an observable physical disability.

ST: Yeah, that's so interesting. Because when I ran into people I hadn't seen in a month or so after my open-heart surgery, I seemed to be automatically asking, "Hey, wanna see my scar?" And there I was pulling up my shirt and proving to the world why I missed the gatherings and the workouts ... because I had open heart surgery. I mean, it's kind of like I'm proud of it, or to your point maybe I'm looking for validation. People don't believe me sometimes unless they look at a really gnarly 12-inch scar and think "Fuck, that guy went through a lot."

JP: This is what my life's like. I can't just snap my fingers, and you see what I see for a second and then I snap them again. You go, "Whoa! That was a trip!" You have to fully believe what I tell you, that I cannot see anything in the middle of my central vision. It's all blurred out. But there's no way you can fully empathize with my situation unless you are legally blind, or your vision is really bad. Some folks are like, yeah, without my contacts I can relate. Okay. Then you can kind of empathize. But once you put those contacts on or wear those glasses, you're able to drive, I'm not.

Prescript: On June 5th, 2024, I underwent open heart surgery to replace a failing ascending aorta and fix a leaky aortic valve. The cardiac issues caught me by surprise and to date, there is no identifiable cause, though ongoing research suggests a variety of cardiac pathologies in long-time endurance athletes. I knew the rehab was going to be tough. But still, there was nothing that could've prepared me for the months that followed. I tried to keep a log of my experiences and feelings, but that task began to feel forced and tedious; I just wanted to forget the entire episode and move on. I couldn't, though. And I didn't; there were just too many telling details. It was almost as if I was being offered a bunch of life lessons. And all I had to do was have my chest cracked, my heart stopped and ask another human to touch it. Below is a random sampling of entries from my log.

Heart to Heart

> *"For long months of days and weeks Ahab and anguish lay stretched together in one hammock rounding in mid-winter that dreary, howling Patagonia cape; then it was that his torn body and gashed soul bled into one another."*
>
> —H. Melville, *Moby Dick or the Whale*

Dateline 6/11/2024. La Jolla, California, Scripps Memorial Hospital Prebys Cardiovascular Center

The thing about hospitals is few of us want to enter them. But if you are a patient in need of serious healthcare and are interned for a few days or a week or more, you are afraid of leaving them.

When I landed in the ICU the afternoon of my surgical aorta and aortic valve replacement (SAVR-only the military has more acronyms than the medical field), I counted 16 tubes and wires somehow connected to me. Some went to veins, some plugged into arteries, two went into my lungs. There were iPod-sized boxes with wires that had a direct pathway to my heart. I looked like one of those experimental versions of a human robot.

And the best part was a secondary wrist band next to the one that held an inclusive bar code indicating such minutia from my social security number to my 6th grade Biology test scores. It was a bright yellow loop with the words "FALL RISK" emboldened in black. As of this post six days later, most of the tubes and wires have left my side but I'm hoping to keep my "FALL RISK" band until next winter's big surf season.

If you've never vacationed in an ICU, I have one suggestion. Don't. But if you have the fortune and are even of questionable faculties, look around, feel the energy, the awe of technology, know there is a reason the staff wake you every 15 minutes to take vitals, draw blood, push meds. Docs, nurses, and staff are not there to make you comfortable; they are there to keep you alive.

According to my surgeon, Dr. Sam Baradarian, the procedure went well. He and his team successfully paused my heart, replaced the torn and tattered parts, restarted the engine, and told me, "Now, it's up to you." Which sounds a bit dramatic. But during those dark and lonely hours, usually late at night when you can't sleep, you can't dream … all you can do is take a breath in and then let it out, in those unconscionable hours, you begin to appreciate the people who gave you the gift of life, who've sacrificed studied, and followed their warrior's heart path down a rabbit hole that has become a morass of healthcare obstacles. These are the frontline fighters of disease and pathologies and every example of trauma from childhood boo-boo to decapitation. They are giving you another chance. Then it's up to you.

As I lie there, counting ceiling tiles in the ICU, I ponder these circumstances, these earthly gods poking and prodding my body. Why am I here? What breath landed me in a place for sick people? How soon can I go home? Will I ever be completely normal again? Should I feel guilty for living what I thought was a healthy life? I know the blame-game will work against me but I'm human and I want revenge. But who? My parents for passing down a less-than-perfect gene? The man in the mirror for thinking that endurance training will keep him free of cardiovascular disease. And then the rational thought returned and Nicole the Night Nurse came in to check on me.

Trying to make conversation, if only to take my mind off the pain, I asked how many patients she was looking after on that evening. "Only you," she said, "my job is to keep you alive." And that's when my rehabilitation began; when I morphed the guilt and blame and anger to appreciation if not acceptance. I have taken risks in my life. But by the grace of God and modern science, I was still here. And I had this funny thought about risk and science. If you want to do something very risky and exciting, go on a trip to a developing country and end up with a staph infection. Many times, your return ticket can only be punched by fortitude, luck, and divine intervention. Or you die in a developing country and your heirs will pay bribes to the officials to bring your body home. The world may be full of every type of healer but when you are very, very sick, would you rather have advanced robotics, experienced medical staff, and measured pharmacology carving out your tumor? Or an ageless psychic shaman anointing you with elderberry garlic paste?

Dateline 6/9/24.

A lot of patients end up loving their surgeon; the savior that returned them to life. Why wouldn't you? I didn't fall in love with Dr. Baradarian. No, I went one better: I respected him. I know that is one of my many essential flaws as a human—this lack of respect for some (well, actually a bit more than most) people I encounter. I know this can be awkward and certainly not fair. But I make people earn my respect. And if you make the list, I have a kidney for you if you need one.

After I was transferred to a regular floor and room, I began to meet the most amazing patients and staff. On one of my first forays outside to my room, I had my wife, my nurse, and a nurse's aide riding shotgun on my walker-assisted jaunt across at least 20 yards of tiled hallway. Feeling like a explorer, I stopped at a 7th story window and gazed out on a world that I hoped would accept me back, even make me better for my Ahabian suffering. A fellow heart surgery patient saddled up next to me; similar tubes flowing out of him like tree branches.

"You ever gonna take this for granted?" He mumbled.

"If I do, it will only land me back here again."

Reduced to the common denominators in life, we speak in levels—pain, mobility, family, and deviance. Speaking across a narrow dark space, it seems odd to me that I am having this kind of conversation with a person I just met and will never see again. He's a strong guy, almost mountain man-ish. If we were in a war together, he'd have my back. And I'd buy him a strong drink.

In the afternoon, the room is quiet. Outside it is cool, almost winterish for a San Diego June. My healing nurse moves my bed next to the window, brings pain pills, fresh pillows, and a menu. The coastal marine layer has darkened the sky and for the moment, the halls are still. I lay there and thought again, the bone-level pain moved just out of center for the time. When did you do that last? Just lie on the floor and let your mind wander. Ideas might start out in the world, get filtered through reading and research, maybe even put into play. But they are catalyzed in the rare quietude of the cool afternoons of our lives; those soft moments when we allow ourselves to be taken down and taught by some teacher who waits across the room, the sound of her steps imperceptible. The white noise of modernity stands as an aural barrier to what potential lies inside. There is a time for rock and a time for Bach but what is missing is what exists in the rents and seams of our nervous reflection.

The thing with open heart surgery is that, as much science and training and preparation goes into having your chest cracked and your heart stopped in hopes of fixing the broken parts in and around this amazing piece of God's engineering ... you never know the end results. People have spoken of changes in personality, taste buds, and choices between Ford and Chevy trucks. And there are setbacks.

My only other major surgeries were replacing my worn-out hips; mostly linear procedures related to the ship-in-a-bottle procedures required when you are dealing with the heart. My first setback happened when I went back into a-fib on day three post op. As an athlete, you identify your enemy, know his strengths and weaknesses, study the rules, and go into battle. Going back into a-fib, for me, and even though it happens at least 30% of the time (over the one to six months post op) in my type of surgery, it was frustrating. Unfair. Disrespectful.

The following days, things became more stable. I was becoming more accepting and a part of me emerged that I didn't know what to do with. I'd always wanted to be that Marlon Brandon character from the 1953 film, *The Wild One*. Brando, as motorcycle rebel, Johnny Strabler, is asked by the town sheriff what he and his marauding gang are rebelling against as they take over the Northern California town of Hollister.

Stabler replies, "What you got?"

I didn't want to come through this thing without an edge. But I wanted to get through it. And I asked myself what I had.

Dateline 6/12/24.

What I remember about that first week home from the hospital is sleeping. I'd sit in the back yard in a big chair, put my feet up, pull my hat down and nod off. A friend who had similar surgery had told me that I'd look back on that first month fondly and remember how, amidst the pain and struggle, there were moments of calm and serenity. Going through a rehabilitation from anything is like that: there are times when a kind of peace and acceptance sneak in as you feel the world has conspired against you. At night, I didn't sleep as well as I did sitting in my backyard at noon. But on average, I'd log 10 to 12 hours each day in slumber. That's the time the body does its best work in repair. Knowing I'd probably never have the luxury of this much daily sleep ever again, I'd pull my hat down and embrace the nothingness.

Dateline 6/14/24.

There are moments during the rehab process when you might wonder what's left when it's all over. Not just the emotional leftovers but physical scars. Once all my bandages came off and the tape was removed, I looked at the 10-inch zipper in my chest. It was still red, raised, and telling. And I had no real investment in the final aesthetic outcome. But I'd seen the result of my surgeon's work on a few friends and to be honest, the thin red line had faded along with some of the memories of how it got there. It was mildly amusing when I'd run into others who had open heart surgery and even as near-strangers, they'd pull up their shirt, show me the scar, and say welcome to the Zipper Club. I think I'll do the same in the future.

Dateline 6/16/24.

Rehab is nothing but healing. Eight days after surgery I'm home and embracing this idea. My rehabilitation is measured in houses, the number I can walk to on my block. The first few days I can get to the fourth house on the cul-de-sac. The next day I got greedy and went for eight houses. But that, along with dehydration, a huge hunk of salmon, and a half bottle of strong IPA sent me into an arrhythmia ... a kind of purgatory for the patient in cardiac rehab. But over the next week, the progress was linear, measured, and clear. Ten houses; two full streets, and then the coveted circumnavigation of the entire block.

Too often we hear the cliché "It's the small things." But in my case, it was relevant and true. And at three weeks post-op I threw caution to the wind and rode my bike around my neighborhood. No Tour de France champion could be happier. This was a very big, small thing. My surgeon had said the only way I could fuck it up was to allow the suture site to get infected or to fall before the six-to-eight-week window and re-fracture the sternum. What could go wrong, I thought as I peddled the rusty beach cruiser up and down my street like a six-year-old on Christmas morning.

Dateline 6/23/24.

The pain in my sternum is intense. Mostly at night, I hear the electric saw cutting that boney plate in half and allowing access to the heart. I know there is permanent wire holding it together. I know the pain will subside. And I think *all this is temporary* and I am a lucky son-of-a-bitch to have found and treated this pathology. But right now, it hurts like hell. I'm maxed out on acetaminophen at 4,000 mg in a 24-hour period and for some reason, I was sent home from the hospital with no narcotics (the good shit). Maybe it was a push-back from the Oxycontin crisis. Maybe it was an oversight. The only thing that mattered to me was that I couldn't get to sleep and couldn't heal and improve and go back to work and go running and surfing and throw my grandkids into the air unless I found a way to make the pain go away. That's when I remembered I had a secret stash of Percocet left over from a previous surgery some years ago. That's the funny thing about the pain part of rehab: in your mind, the short-term matters more than the long term. At least for a while. I wasn't worried about getting hooked and having to go into rehab from narcotics addiction. I just wanted to file an edge off the red-hot poker that was branding my chest. Ten minutes after taking 5 mg. (one pill of the good shit), I was living the dream. Better living through chemicals.

Dateline 6/24/24.

As part of my rehab, I'm given the chance to attend a session where you are monitored and encouraged to move your arms and legs in a cardiac rehab training facility. But if you're a impatient person like me, the only thing you are training is your tolerance for some very easy exercises. That's the ex-pro athlete talking, of course, and the nurses and support staff are using established cardiac rehabilitation practices to guide you. On several occasions, when the physiologist moved over to another client on the treadmill or exercycle, I turned up the speed and resistance. And the nurse watching my pulse and blood pressure on a remote monitor marched out and said, "Mr. Tinley, the reason you're here is that likely you thought more was better. If you want to screw up your recovery, go somewhere else. I don't want anyone dying in my lab." I've come to like this part of the rehabilitation process: listening to experts. Following their advice is a bit more challenging. But this was no Nurse Ratched. I trusted my advisors and was not to be denied.

Dateline 6/27/24.

It's been three weeks, and I can sense the honeymoon ending. Where family and friends would stop by on a regular basis, the parade was slowing. Some stayed just the right amount of time, bringing a pre-made meal and a sense of humor while others wanted to "fill me in" on all their summer adventures that I'd missed. A few, awkwardly, didn't know what to say. They meant well but just kind of stood and stared at me in my backyard chair. And so, I'd pull my hat down and pretend to sleep until the point was made. How others handle your rehab might have something to say about how *you* are handling it. I was surprised at the outpouring of support, and in some ways also confused about the silent ones. Generally, I'm sure the counselors will argue that the more support for the patient of rehab, the better. But at times it's interesting if not stressful to try and find the right words. Just a few months before my surgery, I was talking with a dear friend who is dying of pancreatic cancer. The best I could do was, "This fucking sucks, we'll miss you." Which is, of course, more about living than the dying.

Dateline 6/30/24.

I'm three and a half weeks post op and am reasonably sure I will come out of this episode as good as new. But there's always a part of you that thinks, "As long as I have to go through this shit, why not try to come out better than new?" I think a change in venue will help. So, I fly to the mountains of Colorado and set up camp at a little apartment at 6750 feet above sea level. For a variety of reasons, I've had this escape route on my yearly schedule for over forty years. I came back to my home near the beach, renewed and ready for the fall semester. I've dodged some of the summer crowds and told everyone that Labor Day is my favorite holiday. My surgeon said I was "mostly safe to fly." When I asked him about the "mostly" part he told me to book an aisle seat. To know where the AED was stashed.

Everything was going to plan. I was riding my bike, hiking the trails, swimming in a secret pond, and generally doing a decent job of forgetting that I was supposed to be rehabilitating from open heart surgery. But I'd sort of forgotten about the altitude part. I'd successfully triaged out the pain and misery of my early post-operative weeks in an effort to reconnect with normalcy. And the mountains came calling so I kept up my training between six and nine thousand feet. Until I kept slipping into atrial fibrillation, an arrhythmic condition where the atrium "flutters" causing a decrease in cardiac output, elevated pulse, shortness of breath, and generalized anxiety. The treatment was to sit on the couch; something that, believe it or not, I'm not very good at. The cure is a slow, easy, methodical, and intelligent return to fitness. Something else I am not good at.

Dateline 7/14/24.

It's almost six weeks since they sliced me from stem to stern and I'm smelling the barn. I want to be as fit and fast and hip and groovy as I was a few years ago. Hell, who doesn't? That's one of the hidden problems with extended rehabilitation: a more youthful and vibrant person creeps into your image of what you will look and feel like when the healing is done. Though some people are satisfied if not happy with getting the simple things back—lack of pain, mobility, a reasonable appearance, a degree of sight or hearing—others want more. As if we are taking revenge on our bodies for failing us and now—during our rehab—are demanding the clock is rolled back for our troubles.

I was trying to be reasonable with my requests but the elephant in the room screamed, "Hey knucklehead, your physiological greed is why parts of your heart failed!"

August 21st, 2024

Well, I got what I deserved. Several days before there was a return to running. Even though I was only slugging out 12-minute miles on the treadmill for up to two minutes at a time, I felt like Steve Prefontaine winning the national 10,000-meter title in front of his Hayward Field crowd. So, I ran the next day … a little bit more. And the next day, a bit quicker and on an incline. And then my heart refused to cash checks that my mind was writing. Into the atrial flutter I fell and stayed in that compromised place that lowers your cardiac output and raises your anxiety for three days. Finally, on Friday 8/21, I went into the hospital, got loaded up with Propofol (Michael Jackson's drug), and was cardioverted back into sinus rhythm. Waking up, you feel sleepy but rested and energized because now your heart is beating as it's designed to.

A friend of mine stopped by that night and said, "Dude, if your summer was a fish, I'd throw it back for you."

Mid-September 2024.

There are signs that some degree of normalcy is returning. But as the Canadian singer/songwriter Bruce Cockburn argued, "The trouble with normal is that only gets worse."

Where to now, St. Peter?

SECTION 3:

THE REHAB OF LIFE'S STRUGGLES

Introduction

When I think about what *rehabilitation* means to the Everyman, the Regular Joe or Mary who's had some success in life but perhaps equally, gets their ass handed to them, I think that rehab is not a place, an event, or a medical procedure. Rehab for most people is trying to make the best of something that, wrongly faced, could make the burden of living greater than the joys of human existence. Rehab is getting out of bed, making it to work on time, remembering your spouse's birthday, fitting into jeans, and affording one week's vacation on the Jersey Shore. Approached from the perspective of the inevitable, rehabilitation takes the form of something between survivalism and the certainty of need for pleasure. If you are human, you will be faced—more or less—with the vagaries of war. You might be drafted, maimed, killed, displaced, or debilitated. Or you might be slightly inconvenienced by travel delays and a rise in the costs of imported goods from (enter war-raved country here). If you are human, you will face—in some way, shape or form—the loss of love, freedom, health, and your best friend. If you are lucky, your parents will pass away old and happy and asleep in their comfortable bed, holding hands and appreciating their good fortune. But maybe not. You will see and feel and be humbled by death as many of us who took the COVID-19 pandemic seriously were. Those of us as first responders perhaps not because we wanted to be affected but because we HAD to be affected. But chances are, you will survive and with any luck or effort, you will appreciate Nietzsche's aphorism, "That which doesn't kill you only makes you stronger.

Rehab for many of us is just doing the best that we can.

> *Prescript: During the Vietnam War, every young American male had to negotiate the mandatory draft. Some got out on technicalities, some moved abroad, some went underground, some served. The U.S. government's right to induct expired on June 30th, 1973, less than four months before my 18th birthday. My draft number was 13. Later, I had the great fortune to interact with hundreds of vets returning from theaters of war in 1970s Southeast Asia and in the 90s, soldiers returning from the myriad wars in the Middle East. The following is a fictional look at one vet's rehabilitation. It was based on what I'd seen and felt from those that served and then came back. It was based on what I'd missed and could only imagine.*

That Said and Undone

There's something about the way they hang under the thick midday sun, its rays, asking for nutrients up from the dark blood-earth through the trunk as it sways in the trades, pumping and lifting the sugars through the branches and out toward the thick, fiery fruit. The papayas are always sweeter after the noon sun.

There's only one day at a time down here. And you don't have to worry about being somebody different tomorrow than you were today.

Lita would never pick papayas before the sun pasted its zenith. And even then, she will sometimes wait an extra hour or so; wait until we are just about ready to have our afternoon meal. Then she will smile at me, her sunset teeth and summer hair, a reminder of the place that formed the beauty that lay above and below her quiet history.

She will reach for her reed basket and tell me in her native tongue, purposely imitating my limited Spanish, "Voy para papaya," adding coyly, "the ones shaped like ojos de naranjas." And when I see her return with that woven basket perched atop her long black hair, dancing toward me on the trail in her blue and yellow sarong, the afternoon rain moving in on cue to cool the mid-day heat as the fine, pink sand soaks up the sky like the soft part of a brain soaking up memory, one hand on the basket, the other lifting a plumeria to her nose, well ... I do not think of how I got here or what I had to let go.

It's a strangely comfortable thought to look at a place and feel that maybe, just maybe, you have enough good fortune left in your life to die there; that you've earned the right to do so. But earning has little to do with anything. At least it didn't, in my life.

For many years, I never figured there was any logical sense to it, unless you count random, senselessness, which, I suppose, is a kind of order in and of itself.

Someday I will think of the others, the ones that forgot too soon about what we did, what we were. They're living up on some hill with a new family to keep them out of the tragic ditches of their dreams. I won't regret not going up to see them in real time, pulling them out of a sandy pit, blood finding its way out of new holes in their bodies. That will be them, not me. Just some illogical fallacy framed around a nightmare that began as a childhood game with toy guns. They will have new lives. But old scars.

And all those months on the road I will spend, looking to make sense of what my life was and had been, just so that I could allow it to go forward. Or at least sideways. There will be no obvious order there either, just a wander, a walkabout, an unfolding and unmasking of the hope in life itself. Like Jesus in the desert. Like the desert in itself.

Maybe hope is an illusion after all; it takes you out of the eternal now. I like faith better. It lets you move between *then* and *now* without getting your feelings hurt. Think of hope as a starter kit, like when you get scared and hope you don't get shot. Then you develop the beginning of faith because even if you do catch one in the chest, you believe you have a good shot at living in another world, here inside a new skin or someplace that comes to you while laying your weapons at the altar. That's Faithville, man. And it's gotta' be solid.

It's like sawing soft wood—the blade goes through easily but you're still sawing. And you need a straight line. It's been a few years now, but back then I could never find anything beautiful or uplifting about dying and returning to our maker. I'd heard of immortality. The third-tour guys and religious freaks torching themselves on the corner would touch upon it, but I'd never seen it in the war for real. And I never seen it at a funeral or in a dead body, even when I went looking for it.

What I learned about dying, I learned through staying alive, by accident, not design. By letting myself get too close to the ones that left me. That died. Death on its own taught me nothing. But the process of life bubbles right to the surface when you know that yours or one who you've gotten to know, even admire, that their time is close. Holding your hands inside a buddy's gut ripped open by a frag grenade or IED, pinching off a spurting artery and talking to him just like you were speaking over the backyard fence with your garden hose bent in half to stop the water while you chatted about the game or the new boat he was looking at and lying to him that it was just a flesh wound, that he'd be getting a month in some rehab hospital for recovery, that lucky son of a bitch, and about this one place that you knew of where the girls were soft and went down as smooth as the sake, and to hang in there, "Cuz it was nothing the docs couldn't fix," and medics were on the way and they'll give him some morphine and he'd feel better, now close your eyes and get some rest but before you do look at me, now look at me god dammit, don't you fucking go and die on my ass 'cuz we got stuff to do back in the world. Now, look in my eyes … you hear me, mother fucker? You owe me!

You keep lying to him until the soft sounds of heart's footsteps don't echo in sync with the thump-thump of the Hueys and he won't keep his eyes open and your criteria for falsity and truth is further cultivated by the schizophrenia you embrace like a three-year-old fondling a dead sparrow.

You'll be all right, and then you hold him like you held your mamma did when you got lost in the big store. And he holds you back and whispers words unnamed and unknowable.

Then the son of a bitch is dead gone and for a brief moment, you forget his name but remember his kid's birthdates and the color he planned on painting his Chevy Camaro when he got back.

You go on living, knowing more about life because when he looked into you with those young, scared eyes, he passed along all that he knew and felt and had learnt in-country as a kind of gift that would open on its own accord, on its own time, anyplace but there.

All this he did for you, partly because he could, partly because you would've done the same. All this happened right before that long, deep sigh.

And if per chance, he screamed and called out in some language of the lost or at least the loss that you couldn't respond to, you've had to chase that sound away with every ghost that came back and you purposely, palpably, exorcised them all on the outskirts of towns like Nogales or Santa Fe or Laramie or Durango. Like a rabid dog, you could either shoot them dead or shoo them into the next town. But no more guns please. And so, you bargained and closed your eyes and hoped for the best. Never sure. Cognitive Dissonance, the docs at the VA called it. And you lived with it like a forever rash until one day that three-year old girl opened her hand to offer you the dead sparrow. Only it was a yellow and white daisy. And a map to the Promised Land of DMZ's.

======

Things are good here, though. What happens from day to day still can't be called order so much as rhythm, a natural ebb and flow, a simple existence with Lita, our daughter, Makoi, the local villagers and our immediate world on this island off the coast of South America. An archipelago for the wounded of soul, Father Damien could come step off the copra supply boat with a handful of faceless and fingerless and nothing would matter. War is just a different kind of flesh-eating disease.

An island. Ironic, but not really. I would've thought I'd end up in a more stable spot, geographically speaking, assuming I didn't end up under the ground. Most of the islands in this region are old though, they aren't fluid and moving and spewing new earth out of their highest peaks. But they haven't been aged at the hands of modern man either. This is young adult land—old enough to have an idea of where it's going but not grown cynical from the journey. I thought about the island's teen years, when fiery molten worlds moved villages and added to the shores, leaving a steaming mist as it mixed with the sea and the sulfur hung in the air for weeks, sighing. But things down here don't follow chronological times. People grow sideways before growing up.

The fluid earth: that must've happened a long time ago. But even then, people were fighting over something—land or religion or politics or women. The earth must've been a violent place to live during those six days when God was the GC or the sixty million years it took for the world to evolve organically. Either way, there are days I'd argue that it got worse as soon as man came around.

Before I left the war I was gonna go and talk to one of the guys from the 101st Airborne. Tell him I'm going off the grid, going south. Flyboys have a different perspective. He'll probably say once you come back from the Nam or Korea or any war, don't matter what you do with your life 'cuz they ain't never gonna' let you back on. Not completely. He'll say I wasn't the only one who opened doors on themselves; tell me to go forget about quadrants and little squares with borders that you only know about when you pass a sign or a checkpoint. He'll say the great blue world scattered with green dots; that's more like the beginning of it all. Personally, he'll say, there's places most guys ain't looked for under their pillow.

I'll respect him for that but agree that I'd likely be happier in a place with no certifiable history of the kind that I was used to; the kind that had sent us to do unconscionable things for their premeditated good.

The shadow men. 'Cuz like the song says, I ain't no fortunate son.

<hr>

Fighting for your sanity is a different war all together; a sustained, protracted jungle warfare that somehow seems at place within the vines and branched synapses of your brain. But it's not like you can go to safety behind your own lines for R and R. You don't even carry it. It carries you. There's *no peace with honor* bullshit. Only a form of mutual détente.

I will conclude that it was all irrevocably pre-determined. Maybe not genuine in my reflection of the moment, but truthful in the end because at some point, and I don't know exactly when, I stopped looking for answers in my past and decided to let them find me in the present. I stopped fighting and was given the medal of *Who-Gives-a-Fuck*. Let the devil's germs and guns and concerns move in the front door and out the back. More Buddha, less Beowulf.

Those ideas live in me now, like an ageless lap dog, forever loyal and available. Life down here is one long poem where I can bring up the ghosts one at a time and write them a shape, shake hands and then wait for the trade winds to blow them away. They still visit but they don't stay.

Life, if we cut it up, it dies in the process, killing those around us too, plain as day. Killing taught me that. Not fluffy bunny rabbit moments. Not rainbows and unicorns.

Yet some nights when I lie in our hammock and the sweat comes beading little islands of salt on my body-map, I'm injected by the jungle sounds and smells, and am tripped to Hueys and Tet and Khe Sahn and Sweet Jane and inventing separate realities when I needed them and an enemy wearing pajamas that played prairie dog with the rest of us who are walking around in the sun and the rain stuck halfway between Kumbaya and the Eve of Destruction. Simple grunts. Superior technology, my ass. Kids from poor cities trying to find a way up through the choking seaweed of urban streets and domino-theory McCarthyism; we'd have been better off in black pajamas and a real reason to kill.

But then I close my eyes, weave my arms and legs through Lita like all those vines of my past and let my mind take me where it will. As I fall asleep or go a few rounds with Morpheus, our hearts flow together like water until I can't tell where I end and she begins and the last sound I hear is her own humming and my submission to the white noise of the world. It's the sound of a long deep sigh.

Someone once argued that fear turns men into coyotes, poisons their hearts. I guess that whoever lit my flame of fear certainly has the right to blow it out. Way down here, I won't be afraid of the pain. When it gets too heavy to lift, brush aside or takes on a new disguise, I can burrow my lined and leathered face deeper into Lita's brown-skinned breasts, her innocence acting like some sort of filter, some South Pacific dream catcher that takes the hurt and softens it or gives meaning to the nightmare stepping on it.

Yep, the closer I get to tomorrow, the further I get from yesterday.

═══

I've come to believe that the best stories always begin at the end. And they begin with a dream. Dreaming this way always helps to thaw the sea that has frozen around my heart. I believed in its truth and its lies as much as I did the truths and lies of Saigon and Hanoi that tried to swallow me then back in Vietnam. Or those younger bastards sucked into Iraq and Cheney's weapons of mass destruction. All of us, trying to put war behinds us—Ukraine, Gaza, Iran … hell your own backyard—dreaming of only 40 days and a wake up and a bird back to the World. The blood of amnesia will be on all our hands.

One day I will emerge unvanquished. Forty days, forty nights, forty fuckin years and a wake up.

And someday, God willing, every vet will get their island and their Lita, their manifest turned destiny. No longer will the memory banks want to foreclose on you before papers are drawn and quartered.

Someday, we won't be afraid of the dark. We will learn how to cry again.

Only forty days and a thousand nights from my grid-less land of papayas and no telling one day from the next. I can pull a straight forty; I deserve to live another four decades. I am Jesus in the desert. Tempt me. Go ahead.

This is where I begin. I can feel it now in the words scribbled on the back of a dessert menu from the Continental Hotel in Saigon.

War, I've done. The rest will jump off the screen in Technicolor; brilliant, edible but never as dangerous.

Prescript: As our firstborn went off to college, it dawned on me that every parent suffers a kind of loss when their children leave home. The rehabilitation process varies, of course, by every family. For some, perhaps the dotting mother, there is a deep fracture in their identity as if a relocation of a child signals a small death of self. For others it is a worthy and necessary step toward maturation and adulthood. When we dropped our daughter at an out-of-state university dorm, my wife couldn't even kiss her at the door, the sadness was just too stifling. As an over-protective father, I wanted to get a job at the college just to be close enough to keep the horny boys away. It all worked out, of course and our daughter was closer and smarter and more savvy within three semesters. Thinking back, my wife and I had to adjust to having one less child around the house, one less mouth to feed, one less person to hide the TV remote from but not one less person to love and protect. We were just doing that remotely. Recently, I've begun to wonder if my mother felt the same way when I moved out at 16 years old, needing to be free of a sometimes-heavy-handed stepfather. Probably not when she had another six kids in the house to drive her crazy. Still, losing a family member, whether to their death or relocation or some stupid misunderstanding, requires a kind of rehabilitation. The following was my attempt to make sense of the feelings her mother and I were experiencing.

Red Tide

Your room looks no different. I stand at the doorway, standing sentinel to the past when Barbie dolls stood in corners awaiting your return; a change of tiny clothes; a ride in the plastic Corvette across the magic carpet of your bedroom floor, wind in their hair from your small, tidy-pursed lips. Their future drove in sync with yours—all wide open.

A light leaks out of the closet, and I walk over to turn it off, never remembering when you were old enough to sleep without that luminous lifeguard.

Your room looks the same—unkempt, unruly—like you had just rushed out to meet your friends at the curb, embarrassed for them to see me dressed like them, unkempt, unruly, dangerously close by accident to camo-fatigue and Rasta-colors.

I can still smell your perfume, your peppermint incense and your youth. It hurts to breathe that deep, to smell that far into the past.

Your room is a place I love, with its Starbucks-colored walls and chambered waterbeds and dry-wilted prom corsages. I love every carpet stain that I scolded you for and remember the Big Red Spot that must've been ink or wine or blood and see the circular replacement of newer carpet as if the groundskeeper has changed the holes on the greens. I laugh, knowing that the ink on this page is me bleeding our loss, your gain, pried open by red grapes and time. I wipe away a tear so as not to leave salt on the past.

Your room still has pictures of you and me. I wonder if your dorm room walls, I will grace. I wonder if some college-guy will come in and ask, "That your old man? Can he still surf?" And what will you say to him, this guy, this kid, really, who represents all that lies beyond the horizon while your mother and I watch the sun go down.

In your room, we still exist together. There is tangible evidence: more pictures, wet towels for us to pick up, the lost portable phone, the Eagles CD I've been looking for this past month. In your room the memories are fresh as your child-skin and deep as a knife wound. They are embedded in the sheets you asked me to cuddle you in after a nightmare, entrenched in the blankets that you puked on the first time you stumbled home drunk. Memory's chisel could not re-shape the sweet ghosts that came to us here.

I move across the floor of your room. You've been gone, off to the big city for less than a day and your phone rang. I answer and tell the caller that you've gone out, unable to say that you've moved out. Unable to tell the truth, I descend into myself. For I had let a pathetic fallacy slip into my mind—my baby girl would never grow up, would never leave. There is a large white space between then and now. I can't enter it or reason with myself across it. You've gone away to college, gone away to school. It doesn't matter because you're not here.

The bed in your room is still unmade and I laugh because you are like me— reasoning that a bed will only get messed up each night. Why make it look good for no one else to see? But I see it and pick up your pillow, holding it to my ear like a seashell a long way from the beach, hoping to hear you call out to me at three in the morning, "Daddy, Daddy, I'm scared. Can you sleep in my bed?" But memory and the rosy tint of nostalgia are no longer a refuge or a shelter from what must be. Our time with you living with us must be the last true currency of any value. It is sacred, immutable. How selfish of me to want more?

This is how life must change—not one moment or one day at a time but one child-turned adult, one realization that, as Nietzsche said, "Without self-division there is no self-analysis." And so I analyze my angst and watch as it pings and caroms around your room, missing your closet still filled with shoes, your desk piled with things I think you must need but know that you have six of because we bought you four, skipping over the bookshelf with your friends, Seuss and Chopin and Woolf and Porter and Dickenson and DVDs of foreign films that your first boyfriend enjoyed and you sat through with him. And finally, my loss comes back and lands right where it started—in my own pity. It's a place where my nerve endings dance and dangle and finally explode in the realization that all of it was our pleasure, our privilege to raise a child like you.

That summer day when the lightning nearly struck us in Colorado and you refused to leave the house for a week, that time when you crashed your car six days after you had earned your driver's license, that time when your friends couldn't wake you up in the morning and we spent two days in the hospital knowing the OD was, like most adolescent mistakes, not some badge of finality but a right to fuck up, to look in the mirror at eighteen or twenty-eight or fifty-eight and know that you found your center by dancing on your edges. Those are the exacting times that define my years with you as a child, the times that you were my teacher.

I suppose it is the gentle quietness of the room that begins to meld the past with the future, transferring what was with what might be. It stands in contrast to your younger brother's room, still pulsing and beating with the vulnerability of teenage catharsis. I imagine how I might alter the room, maybe dolly it up for guests or turn it into some studio-type cave for the music and art I think will shield me from remembering your seventeen years in this upstairs corner with a view of the neighborhood streets you drew hop-scotch squares on.

But that wears off slowly, like Novocain, and the cloak of self-deceit is replaced by the reality that maybe you'd like to return to your Pee-Chee folder set, nod politely to your dusty Barbies and chorus of carpet stains; that you'd rather come home for Thanksgiving or for good and face not a furniture-smashing, gun-pulling reunion but slip simply and quietly for a day or a year back into that hallowed brilliance of familiarity. I'd like to think that when you come home and set your suitcase in the middle of the kitchen floor and are pulled like blood to your heart, by the moon's gravity back up to your room, you will lie on the crumpled sheets, smell the sandalwood candles and the fabric softener and see that nothing, really, has changed. Know that then, and forever, as long as you'd like—it is a home.

I can play the wounded vet, a selfish veteran of absence. But not very well.

Screw Thomas Wolfe's notion. Come Thanksgiving we could spill red wine and laugh at the funny shape on the floor. It will go away, as will you, but return, another bottle made better with age; not just time and tide but bound by blood.

Call soon. I won't touch a thing.

Prescript: The COVID-19 pandemic signified perhaps the greatest rehab opportunity for humans to fix ourselves, to do better all the way around than any time since WWII. It was such a moving target though, that making sense of it on paper was risky at best. When we came up for air in the spring of '22, I tried to reflect on the past eighteen months. And even now, some years hence, I wonder why we couldn't hang on to but a few of the silver linings. The pandemic of 2020-2022 was for some the hardest thing they'd ever faced. Thousands of health care professionals leaving their jobs because, as one nurse said, "I just don't want another person dying in my arms." For others it was perhaps a mild inconvenience. While we were in the throes of the lockdown in spring 2020, along with the suffering I noticed some beautiful things unfolding: families spending more time together, a radical reduction in global greenhouse emissions, a spike in societal creativity, people consuming less, sharing more. Recycled bicycles. And I wondered what the world would be like on the other side. Would we just forget and move back to our old habits? Could we carry some of the positive effects forward?

There is no denying that we are different now than we were when COVID was at its peak. But I feel that the jury is still out on if those differences are good, bad, or just … different. Maybe some forms of rehabilitation take not months or years to unfold but decades. This was my response one morning when I realized my job working on the beaches of Del Mar, California was focused on keeping people OFF the beach.

Dear Universe:

I woke up this morning at the crack of nine and focused on the flattening curve of my over-rested spine. From the far shore of the living room, the TV rang the day's stats—another dozen here, another thousand there—real people suffering and profiting and striving and living and dying. Just making the most of the least.

Life as we knew it was not.

The conditions that pre-existed mostly in the minds of thinker/planner types— the deep theorists who considered heavily a world that the rest chose not to think about—had come to their fruitful end. *Pre-existing conditions* now meant everything from bank relationships to hypertension to ICU proximity. All the while, network pundits chirped away from their ideological nests while the country's best pens had gone strangely silent. Where to now, Joan Didion? John Stewart?

We had simultaneously entered a world of medical catch phrases and global focus. Are you asymptomatic or a super spreader? Are you an index patient subject to contact tracing or on lockdown due to immunosuppression? Not since 1941 has Earth been so single-minded in its attempt to solve the ultimate transcendent challenge; all the while staying together/apart. Humans are now asked to act humane. Though from a refugee camp called home. Modern society has taught us to live apart and to live together. But the oh-so-close tease of virtuality—like a grandchild's cry when FaceTime kisses fail—worsens the longing for real lips. It is as Camus suggested within the narrative of his 1948 epic, *The Plague*, the utter absurdity of life, the conflict between our quest for existential meaning and the universe's silent answer.

This is without argument, the golden age of the internet and the perfect excuse for declining hygiene. Accelerated relational effects have reached hyper-space. "I thought that I (enter human emotion—here: love, hate, tolerance, ambiguity et al.) you until the fifth week of watching your dark roots fail to find lightness and levity." But with the stroke of a key, we greedily consume each other's real-time virtual image like some cyber-sex deviant from a dime store novel. And nobody but Bill Gates saw it coming.

And in the rents and seams are the comforts: animals returning to claim modern villages lost to fear and quarantine, 80's styled, steel-framed bicycles being hauled to repair shops in mass. "Can you fix this flat? Oil that chain? Anything but another day of my wife's Zumba classes and the kid's Zoom lesson on fractions."

And what about air quality being the best in decades; the Earth cackling in delight as the echoes of feigned regret ping from the pundits.

What had we learned from COVID-19? What more can we expect to hit us like a falling brick or a whisper in the wind? Where to now St. Peter?

And so many living in fear but not know exactly what they feared.

But fear, as someone pointed out, *turns men into coyotes, poisons their heart.* That week when the number of dead Americans from COVID had surpassed the number killed in the Vietnam War hurt me. The universe had done in ten weeks what war had accomplished in ten years.

I fear that we will have learned little; that eighteen months or eighteen years from now, stuck in newer return-to-normal traffic, we will miss those family walks through the neighborhoods, toilet paper hording jokes, talking with anyone who will listen not for the sake of talking or listening but just to feel the deep comfort of F2F communication. I fear that we will return to egregious consumption, will forget to smile and wave, will forget to wash our hands and pray before bed.

I wonder about how our leaders will be remembered, or whether the rigor of science and hard-earned veracity will be run roughshod once again by the shallow and the trite. Marjorie Taylor Greene attacking Anthony Fauci not because she understands or believes in science but because it appeals to her under-educated far right zealots who elected her. I remember fearing a winter rebound of the virus. It was like waking up from a bad dream and being afraid to fall asleep again. Use common sense, we are told, stay the hell away from each other not because you are mean but because you are kind. The final paragraph in Camus' *The Plague* recalls protagonist Dr. Rieux' observation of a joyous town who is claiming victory over the pandemic.

"As he listened to cries of joy rising from the town … Rieux remembered that such joy is always imperiled … perhaps the day would come again for the bane and enlightening of men, it would rouse up its rats and send them forth to die in a happy city."

So, we take both refuge and folly in former President Trump's accidental existential claim that, "it will all just disappear one day."

And what to make of the protesting hordes, the packed churches, beaches, and basements justified under constitutional rights and basic human liberties? I remember a grade school Civics teacher explaining to my 6th grade cohorts that in a liberal democratic republic, freedom only extended to the point where it affected someone else's freedom. Smoking on airplanes and farting in elevators were the samples she used

So much brilliance and ignorance are forced to the surface not by lack of precedence but by levels of preparedness. What South Korea or Sweden did right, or Italy or New York did wrong are mute points. Until it happens again.

That once bitten cliché.

Did you really think ...

The global pandemic was over because sixty-something percent of the American adult population were vaccinated. Did you really think that every country, however developed, numbered or labeled, would share equally in epidemic erasure? No different than America's TP-stampede and the hording of dumb bells, bandwidth, and bleach. Our social, cultural, and economic forces had separated our nation states with relative definitions of winning and losing.

New Zealand may have won some battle with only two new cases reported. But their geographical isolation may have kept them from accessing the vaccine quick enough to stave off an economic recession. Quality of life becomes a negotiable point for all but the deceased. Not quite collateralized, COVID-19 victims simply died too soon.

The pandemic was thus a kind of war where the fallen were too often forgotten in search of forgetting about the day-to-day suffering. And for many, that pointy end of the needle never felt so good.

Did you really think any market-based economy wouldn't come roaring back when it felt safe enough to travel, to shop or to drink beer in public? Trading nations have been in a state of consumption since Dutchman Peter Minuet bought Manhattan from the native Algonquian people for sixty guilders (about $24) in 1626. Capitalism usually finds a way. Why then, would we doubt that an eighteen month uh, *shift* would not foster a renewed desire to buy shit we don't really need? It was simple as re-focusing our discretionary income from a cruise ship vacation to a Winnebago, from a new car to an electric bike and a wine cellar.

Did you really think that a global pandemic wouldn't foster some of the most creative ideas of our time? Wouldn't cause us to stop and appreciate our health and our loved ones and DoorDash? Who doesn't shake their head when a pop-up ad offers to rent you a shelf of smart-titled books to place in your Zoom background? My favorite was the dream merchant who, after having a claimed dream about any of her clients, would decipher the message and send an invoice to the *dreamee* based on the length, power, and resonance of the dream. I could do that job but most of the dreams I have of others, if made public, would land me in jail.

Many of the COVID-19 connections to commerce will remain in our daily lives. Plexiglass barriers, logo'd masks, parking lot dining, door-to-door delivery of anything that a rational or insane person could dream or desire. Every business but the DMV and the house of ill repute has found a way to offer their services via the world wide web. Which makes Russian hackers and multi-taskers very happy. Even modern sports have morphed with the Paris Olympic Organizing Committee announcing that e-sports may be offered in demonstration at the 2028 games. COVID-19, if nothing else, was a giant debutante ball for the nerds of the world.

God bless the geeks living in their parents' basement earning seven figure incomes.

Some of the pandemic's other conventions, it appears, can't leave our lives quickly enough. Ankle touches and elbow bumps, crossing the street to keep fifty feet away from a stranger in the rain, and the impunity of self-forced isolation has already been dismissed. Other mannerisms and reactions remain in negotiation. To sneeze in public is to fire a pistol at the ceiling. To hug a stranger, to spit on the sidewalk, to share an ice cream cone. It's safe to say that flash mobs and crowd surfing are still on hold.

Did you really think that fear wouldn't sustain its effect on the post-pandemic populist? That the hardscrabble nuances associated with pain and suffering wouldn't follow us into a vaccinated world where statistically, one might perish from a common cold or herpes before COVID-19? What perplexes me is the division caused by COVID fear; as if getting really sick for a few weeks, perhaps dying, is considered on the same level as The Man telling you a vaccine is required to enter a Garth Brooks concert? I get the whole agency versus patriarchy thing, I read Orwell and Huxley. For a time, several states including Louisiana, Arkansas, Georgia, and Mississippi were under 35% for an adult vaccination rate. Their message of resistance might be interpreted somewhere between, "The vaccine was developed too fast," to, "I just don't want Big Gov telling me what to do," to the profundities of Bill Gates' mind-control. Still, in consideration that there are thousands of the globally best and brightest working non-stop on our generation's polio, AIDS, and measles, well … given a choice, I'm gonna go with science before sentimentality, Tony Fauci before Fox News. As noted above, in a civil society, personal freedom only extends until it personally fucks up your neighbor's freedom.

And did we really think that love, work, and religion—staples of our social fabric—wouldn't come out the COVID rinse cycle looking different than when we dropped them in the machine? Relationships put to the acid test as we bear witness to each other's dark roots; a constant party to the tedium of their ad nauseam Zoom calls. Jesus, man, can't you go back to the office? Sit in a cubicle? Give the family a break? Ah, but the office is closed and for many, it ain't opening any time soon. Employers, looking at substantial savings in rent, utilities, and bottled water are giving workers much of what they'd asked for—a chance to prove their individual worth, to dress down, to see their kids at lunch … flexibility. And for those who actually *like* their co-workers, there is always Starbucks. Or the grandiosity of unemployment and lessoning vagaries of virtual dating.

And then there is organized religion. In a time when God and spirit and communitarianism were most in need, we bore witness to super-spreader services; some radicalized right refusing to worship from the relative safety of their living room while frontline workers still got sick and died in the name of a for-profit Jesus if not a misanthropic refusal to actually love-they-neighbor by staying six feet from their soul.

But did we really think that true goodness wouldn't rise from mayhem and mistrust? More good deeds were done during the last eighteen months than I've seen in the last eighteen years. The wolf may have been at our door, but we kept good company with him among with all God's creatures.

Where to now, St. Peter?

I suppose we would be foolish to think that COVID-19 is the last pandemic, that modern science and rationality will reign supremely and that Wiley Coyote will finally ensnare that illusive Roadrunner. But modern science has suggested on an empirical basis that global warming will foster further viral development, that the same excuse we've used for fifty years to turn a blind eye to environmental degradation cannot be used to support new and quick fixes to our next pandemic. That science will always and already fix our fuckups. Thirty years from now, Tony Fauci will likely be dead. But the televangelist industry will rock on. And some kid from the Bronx will be busking in a NYC subway, singing, Dylan's *The Times They are a Changing*.

COVID-19 changed our world. That fact is not debatable. But the *how, when, where*, and *whys* of its effect are up for negotiation. It is our hope that COVID-19 was both a shot heard round the world and one that crossed our collective bows; that the pandemic might wake us up to our social and biological shortfalls; that some Great Spirit tapped humanity on the shoulder and said, "Hey folks, here's a chance to do better."

Still, I take refuge in the thought that in my lifetime, never have so many brilliant men and women around the planet cleared their desks for one singular cause grounded in hopefulness. And in the wake of their efforts, discoveries will come never considered part of the COVID crisis. Cures and ideas and notions and goodness and in the small forgotten faces … more hope. And on the other side, figures in Washington or Wisconsin will take credit. *They did something, dammit.* It doesn't matter what but there was healing in just raging at the unseen enemy.

Prescript: I went through a period when dozens of my friends were getting divorced or leaving serious relationships. The two common denominators appeared to be, first, they claimed they didn't really know "that person" any longer, and second, the loss of a partner could be replaced by a deep connection to a natural world. Some of my friends moved to the mountains, others went on long solo journeys. But the great majority just went surfing. It has been a long time since someone broke my heart. But I remember the feelings and the pain and need to stay strong and realize I would get through it. The piece of fiction below reflects the conversations with my friends who were in the thick of ending a relationship. One particular phrase came from my friend John. Going through a divorce not of his choosing, he called one night after surfing well past dark. "The ocean is my new lover now. She will never let me down."

Eros, Poseidon, and Me

> *"Darkness, darkness, be my pillow ..."*
>
> —Jesse Colin Young, singer/song writer

There was no one to call to file the edge off. Or to sharpen it such that I might open a bottle or a book. My dog knew. Buddy swaggered unhurriedly across the room, looked at me with a been-there-it-hurts-like-a-motherfucker-don't-it eyes. He didn't lick me or curl up at my feet. Maybe he knew that I had to fall through the hole in myself. Dogs don't waste your time with empty sympathy.

The pain left only two options. And I knew she would be pissed if the blood stained the new beige 4-ply carpet.

How hard can it be to snatch something real from the ever-fleeting, to do a thing for the thing's sake, to see the rottenness in life but ignore the smell and reach for the broom? How fortunate was I now, as I had been in the past, to have my own Betty Ford Center two blocks away?

I put an old 3/2 mm wetsuit in my backpack, tossed some wax, the rest of some half-hearted bottle and a mushy apple in the front basket. I grabbed the first board out of the rack and tucked it under my arm. I don't remember coasting down the hill on my bike or scrambling down the bluff as the sun left its mark on the hellish day. I couldn't tell you if it was a beautiful sunset or a cloudy dusk. I knew that it was getting dark all the way around, the sea and the sky welding on the horizon.

Buddy stood on the shore and pointed like a bird dog. Strange for a mutt. "Go home. Go home! Ah, well then forget it, suit yourself." I took a bite of the apple and tossed the core into the sand watching grains stick to it like memory to the soft part of the brain. An after-hours gull snatched the lucky find.

I thought I knew her. I was sure. In the end, it was like the others, shadows of potential, possibility smothered by daily silence. Was it me or them?

Paddling out I began to notice things I hadn't before: the way the cold-water seeps in around your knees before your waist, the way the little wake comes off the tip of your board in angular V's, going somewhere, nowhere. I noticed how the shallow spots on the reef created circular boils on the fast-dropping tide, pulling water, energy, and life from its center back into some black hole beneath the surface, a place from which that life and water were born.

There was only one other guy out, one other surfer in the lightest part of the dark hoping maybe for one last toothy wave of a two-hour session. He only needed a ride in, didn't have to worry about being caught from behind.

I paddled right by him, avoiding his stare. Nothing he could say would've made a difference. Maybe he was just out of the joint and hadn't surfed for three years. Maybe he was a trustafarian who surfed every day to avoid the boredom of excess. I turned my head just enough to lift my chin.

"Word," I said.

"Word up," he replied.

He paddled away. I didn't see him leave the water or walk up the path, only heard a dog bark.

Out of the corner a big set started to well up on the outside reef. How far had this wave traveled only to finally release its energy here in six feet of black, kelpie water? Some orgiastic physics would never explain it. I paddled hard, spun at the last minute and dropped in, Rosetta Stone in sync. At the bottom, I laid it over hard and felt the board bite deep into the wave's face. Anger and regret driving me.

I could've done better with her.

The wave in front now, feeling the rocky bottom, standing up, begging to be held like a child bringing home a picture made at school.

"Look, Dad. Look at this picture I made for you!"

Look, son, look at this wave I made for you.

Inside now, an absence of feeling in my heart, there's darkness at the wave's circular core. It's a place of hope and I strain towards a feint pulsing glow, the glimmer of some left-over refracted light off the bluff as I squirt out onto a broad, nurturing shoulder understanding in some small way what Frankl realized after surviving Auschwitz, "What is to give light must endure burning."

Where does wisdom and perseverance like that come from? Can it be applied to relationships?

Paddling back out, I glanced over at a sea lion. He returned my stare with an odd look, as if to say, "I can do that." The ocean could swallow him up and get nothing. He made an obscenely joyous bark. It was a tempting sound.

The sky reflected only blackness now. I surfed by feel, wondering what it would be like to feel the shark's first strike. Pondering what it would be like to die in such novel way, eviscerated by what tomorrow's paper would call, "A killing machine." A line from Melville pops in, "Queequeg no care what god made him shark."

It would be a fitting death.

I sat for a long time and watched the lunar reflection creep over the edge. It was a teasing light. And sometime after midnight that great block of ice that had settled in my chest began to melt. I wanted to believe that shit about truth at first light, but I felt that it was the night, the absence of external fire, the melding of one day into the next that opened the gates. The rain started; loud but soft.

In the beginning she was real. Now she has changed her eye color with tinted glass. Was I creating my truth or rehearsing my death? Was she?

Almost imperceptible at first, I begin to notice it first in the waves I choose and the way I surf them. Then in my relationship with the ocean surface, the way my board sits gently upon this sheet of smooth black ice, the way my hands softly make quiet little circles on its skin.

I cannot see the advancing swell, but I sense something and paddle hard for the horizon, the lower stars blocked by this lump. Harder now, pulling at still water, onward to meet Her. I am a guest, open to invitations and experience.

When she finally comes, it is like no wave I have ever ridden, big but not unwieldy, imperfect in shape and texture, uneven and raw. She carries me gently, but I cannot stand, content to lie prostrate, my face close to Hers.

Following the shelf, I ride until my fins hit the sandy shore and I stay there, motionless, breathing. The moon bends under a passing cloud. A phosphorescent edge of foam is switched on.

I let the match burn all the way through before grabbing my board and walking toward the cliff. My footsteps kick sand into the air.

She is gone now. They are gone. Buddy is there.

I see her older shadow moving in the dark, digging in bent trash cans outside the theater looking for someone new to play her part. We are making choices in the moment; choices that matter, that hurt.

She still carries that edible mayhem in her, dying and living not in the sunrise but in every south wind. I thanked her for the madness and the adventure before saying goodbye to her gentle violence and half-dead eyes.

I've met someone else, I say to myself, tasting the words. *She comes and goes. We are … old friends.*

Walking back up the wet clay trail, Buddy waits for me at the top, laughing, I imagine, at how humans confuse absolution and absolute. I know that surfing and what is left of my life are there now glaring back in the headlights of a passing train.

I am not haunted by Her.

It only took me twenty-five years to get over the loss of my dad when I was fifteen years old. Probably the longest period I will spend restoring my faith in some natural order. But his early death at 40-years-old mutated any organic pecking order.

Any human with a beating heart (and other mammals in the animal kingdom) will have to deal with the loss of a loved one. It might be a grandparent, it might be a goldfish, it might be a spouse of fifty-years, or it might be a favorite dog. The way we grieve that loss can and does have a profound effect on our future lives.

When I finally let my dad go when I turned forty-years-old, I became fascinated with the concept of heroes. How we struggle to make sense of the ones we choose to elevate us. To inspire and guide and loft our spirits. And then fail us. I still believe in the power and relevance of heroes, particularly the ones who earn that title. The essay below was my effort to document my feelings as I emerged from over two decades of grieving.

In the Name of Our Fathers

> *"The hero is always the embodiment of man's highest and most powerful aspiration"*
>
> —Carl Jung

When my son was nine years old, he used to think I could do no wrong. No other father on the block would attempt a 50-50 rail slide on a skateboard or drop into a plywood half-pipe. I was his hero and nothing else in this world made me happier. I wear scars and scabs of skating like a Scoutmaster's badge.

I never doubt these memories. Unlike the clouded sigh of a Disneyland ride, a second-grade English teacher or a first love, all of them tainted and twisted by the unbalancing effects of re-interpreted youth, hormones never factor between a father and a son. Male blood lines are immune to nostalgic whim.

142

As an angst-riddled pre-teen, in the footsteps of his older sister, he had come to ignore me for making him come home before curfew. The inner tumult wells up from another place and another time; the feeling will not be denied. Still, in these days of teenage individuation, I would give him a kidney the same as I'd ask him to mow the lawn.

On those days, I often think back to the time when my own father, just months from dying, would ask me to help around the house. And I try to convince myself that I did. But I was born with his rebel's heart, and it beat defiantly then, as it does now. I would be lying if I said that I'd done all I could for him.

The singer/songwriter, Bob Dylan has said, "To live outside the law, you must be honest." This is the kind of honesty that haunts you all of your days, this striving toward what was and what could've been. To go back and shake that rebel though, and see what truth or consequences fall from his young branches, also may begin to sprout some freedom found in the self-admission.

I began a rough draft of this piece on February 23, 2001. My father would have turned sixty-five that day. He would have been eligible for Social Security and senior discounts at the movies, and no doubt that night we would've toasted his health with a glass of fine cabernet instead of remembering, missing him more than I could write without arcing into high sentiment, my prose taken hostage by the ache of loss. It's an essay that can never be complete, only passed on. Maybe the pain of loss informs our lives more than we can say in words.

He has been dead for over forty-three years now, since I was a cocky, can-do-no-wrong fifteen-year-old with a restless soul. I have long since passed the age at which he died. But I don't feel old, and I don't think that I will die anytime soon. And I'm no longer afraid of dying the way I once was. I don't think so, anyway.

I suppose that it would be a shame if I weren't able to understand and reconcile his untimely death before I pass as well, to know my hero in death as I knew him in life.

There must be a kind of resiliency to letting those you love go … completely. Or perhaps it's tenacity or egoism or just plain luck. I don't know if you can work at it like you might in a 12-step program to combat alcoholism.

====

I would not wish that my father had played a smaller role in my life simply to escape the pain of his dying. I remember when he "procured" an idle ambulance from the sidelines of a football game and took me and my siblings careening through the streets of Orange County, siren blaring, lights flashing. My mother tried to act disgusted. I think of him as an only child, without siblings to fight or to tell scary stories to on a stormy night or to share a tiny bathroom with. He and my mom decided that they were going to have as many as they could make. It was seven and counting when he left us.

I think of him coming home one night from a poker game with the boys, one too many beers involved, and slipping fifty dollars under each child's pillow—in total a big chunk of what he earned in a month. In the morning, he told my mom that we deserved it, even though they couldn't afford the luxury, because "kids deserve surprises."

I think of him smiling confidently at the guard at a posh country club as he drove through the gate, flashing an expired Union Oil gas card. "The only ones you should let see your fear," he would tell us "are the ones who you can trust with it."

He was no saint. He often refused to go to mass with the rest of the family on Sunday because he'd rather go down to the beach and have his own little bull session with his God. Yes, he had faults, imperfections lost to time and sentimentality and selective memory. He'd gained some weight, lost his patience from time to time. Probably didn't wear a seat belt. But he was a good man. And a lot of our own spirit was taken with him. It's hard to break apart a big Catholic family, even if you're a Buddhist.

I find it ironic that I can accept my own eventual death and yet I cannot make sense of his suffering at the hands of a hideous, indiscriminate disease. Urban legend has it that after Buzz Aldrin piloted the lunar landing module of Apollo 11 into the moon's Sea of Tranquility, he had trouble parallel parking back on earth. It's supposed to be easier to deal with other people's deaths, easier on earth than in space. I don't know if this angst belongs to the past or the future. But if my house is burning down, I won't agonize over which room to paint first.

The lucky ones defer the question all the way to the end. I don't imagine they die well, knowing that they are dying, but not why.

Perhaps my career choices were guided by a secret desire to cheat death: lifeguard, firefighter, paramedic, professional athlete, and then, at forty, graduate student. And still the grand prize, Enlightenment, eludes me. My dad was my hero. Heroes aren't supposed to die.

Whose fault is that this death of our heroes? The hero, for being human after all? Ours, for failing to see the inevitable? Who didn't shudder at the sight of actor Christopher Reeve, strapped to his chair? The mechanical breathing machine that kept him alive out of view, perhaps to shield us from any further reminders of our own fragility—our humanness. Reeve looked disarmingly hopeful, wearing his most courageous public face. Where did his strength come from? The cracked vertebrae came by accident, I know. But was the rest of his life an accident? Let alone his untimely death?

Cartoon heroes are immortal. Humans aren't.

"There but for the grace of God go I," you think, and change the channel. If Superman can end up a physical prisoner on wheels and then sadly slip away, if my dad can be snatched from his wife and children at the height of his existence, how safe are we in choosing heroes?

Over time, public figures and athletic icons have survived injury, illness, bankruptcy, and brutal attacks. They have survived disease and war and have tweaked rampant infidelity into the lesser charge of "marital indiscretion." Professional athletes have returned from prolonged periods of slump only to be hailed as the heroic clutch savior who arose from the performative-dead in time to save the world and the playoff season.

The fallen athlete hero is only a season-saving game away from redemption.

There are few narrative themes in popular culture as resonant as the returning but sinful Odysseus, the contrite Prodigal Son, and the self-healed sickly one who now stands as tribal shaman. But perhaps the greatest challenge for the fallen sports hero is to make amends with a sports fandom they have continually deceived over time. This rabid collective of now-jilted followers who stand stupefied at the water cooler holding a Ben Johnson bobble-head or a Marion Jones poster signed, "All the best," are poised and ready for revenge. "How dare you cheat to win," the seething masses ask, while quietly reflecting on their own indiscretions.

The fallen sports hero reminds us up close and personal just how close the link is between the finite reality of our humanness and the myth of the supernatural performer. And in that narrow space between what we believe and what we want to believe, sits a proud defrocked kid named Lance Armstrong from Plano, Texas, surrounded by a fatherless past and a bank of $1200/hour lawyers.

Or witness the morbid circus that followed the death of stock car racing icon, Dale Earnhardt. Five thousand people attended his televised funeral. For a time after his death, kids in preschool were taught to count by reciting "1-2-Earnhardt-4-5-6-7 ... because the number 3 was always Dale's. The guy drove cars at 200 mph for a living, approaching his job no differently than an accountant or an engineer. But he achieved hero status because he did things that most of us can only dream about, shake our heads, nudge our buddies while pointing to the instant replay, "Did you see that?"

Maybe Earnhardt wasn't a hero in the classic sense of folklore: one who commits a selfless act in the service of others. Maybe he was just a very gutsy, talented driver who went over the edge in the regular course of his job. In fact, athlete-heroes may only entertain us with their exploits, impress us with their creative and athletic skills—and yes, their courage—even if it is a diving catch into the grandstands and not a rush into a fiery building. We are tempted to see in athletes, elements of heroism that often aren't really there; our hopes and imagination placing us in the netherworld hotel where even they can check in.

But never leave by the same door.

Maybe the men and women who scale the world's great mountains are heroes, not for their incredible feats of physical and mental endurance but for our perception that they have stepped further from earth than the rest of us. It's that mystical barrier, we believe, between this earth and the one beyond. And since no one has yet gone there and returned to describe it, we worship those who can get close enough to touch it, to taste the fruits of the Great Beyond.

What's it like? We ask. The mountain? No. Heaven.

==

And what about Reeve? He was simply riding a horse—not an especially dangerous activity. He became a celebrity through a combination of playacting, character type, and mass media exposure. He became a hero to millions through the great irony of this tragedy and his courageous fight to find meaning in what his life had become. All Superman had to do was slip into his spandex tights and red cape to save the world. Reeve had to slip into the interior of his very being to save himself.

I suppose that is part of what I still feel toward my father—the fact that I watched him suffer, watched him stoically endure tremendous physical pain as the cancer slowly and deliberately ate him away. But that was not the worst of it. The worst was that toward the end, he knew that he was going; his trim, surf-tanned body of 170 pounds replaced with a jaundiced shell of 130. He knew he had fought the good fight, done everything possible, made peace with his maker. And all he could do was to wait and try to find some meaning in it. There was nothing else to rebel against.

Some mornings now, as I paddle out before the sun, waiting for its warmth, a few waves before work or class to help make the day more palatable, I too try and find some meaning in it. Yet nearly thirty years and three thousand surf mornings later, I'm not much closer to knowing, except maybe to consider that we aren't supposed to know it at all, which is a kind of meaning.

I can't go back and change what I didn't do, how I didn't spend a few more hours every day with him while he was dying. I can't make the memory of my dad any different. It is a futile wish—a wish to extinguish the last embers of guilt. But making today right can help make yesterday seem less wrong. The beautiful pain of memory is by accident, the painful beauty of imagination by design. At least I know I've tried to be more empathetic with the seriously ill.

=====

As we grow older, we begin to discover our parents' deficiencies. We notice their quirks and oddities. The hero becomes human, exposing the circularity of the things like water sucked down in a whirlpool as kids sit and wonder where it all goes.

My dad died before I could notice his odd little quirks, before he put on a few pounds around the waist, before his sideburns turned gray, before he might've voted Republican, before hair started to grow in his ears. He died standing atop that pedestal on which a young son places his father, part man, part myth. That's when the stories began to bring him back. Or at least to keep him from going too far.

Two days before he was diagnosed with advanced thoracic cancer, he had complained of back pain from "one too many games of beach volleyball." My mom handed him two aspirins. My older sister called him "soft." He picked up the aspirin and threw my sister in the pool.

I'd watched him surf that last healthy day, embarrassed; my parents were invading my teenage space. But secretly I wanted to go up to my friends and scream in their ear, "Did you see my dad's last ride? The dude is three times our age and rips!"

As I age, that is the image that grows stronger in my mind, gradually displacing the images of him weak and withered. That is what I want and must hold onto—a single image of a strong, proud young man, regally perched on the tip of his board, arching across large blue waves, white teeth smile, lighthouse visible.

If I hold that one image tight enough and close enough, all the bad ones fade. It is not easy, one moment of his heaven doing battle with eighteen months of our hell. The numbers work against you, but you have your heart on your side. In the end, that has to be enough.

═══

And just how do heroes come to be? Is it they who follow their hearts, or is it us, the adoring crowd who want to place them in a category that we can strive toward, admire and emulate? Once the hero hears the call to adventure, he will suffer if he denies it more so that he will suffer in the struggle to greatness. We know this from both myth and experience.

But then, as we watch them slip and fall, victims of time, tide and fashion, they still return to us with the knowledge of having lived a hero's existence. Not often do we embrace them for their wisdom. Not often do we glimpse into the darkness from which they have emerged, that place where our metaphysical fear resides.

And then, in that clouded circularity, the hero again becomes victim, disposed of by a disposable society. His foe no longer dragons or evil forces or even age and miles of hard road. It is us, discarding that which we've used. Their declining beauty and achievement remind us of our own morality and that the beauty of our youth will soon be replaced with our own truth of loss. Our own mortal decline, hair in the ears and all.

Where we can check out but never leave.

Most of us die too young or too old. At some point we must realize that on some grander scale, life is indeed short and our ego-filled existence utterly insignificant. We try to pull ourselves up by making love, making money, making the grade; all the while making less and less time to face the fact that we can't do it alone. And when we can't, we look to others to do it for us—our heroes. In one way or another, we are all defined in others. This should be celebrated, not considered a weakness.

Sometime after his career had ended, as his health began to fail, the great Mickey Mantle was spotted by a reporter in a hotel lobby, sitting alone next to a window, listening to the rain bounce off the large, clear panes. When the reporter approached, Mantle held up his hand and said softly to the man, "Listen. It sounds just like applause, doesn't it?"

A hero is born with a Warrior's Heart, the need to be needed. Sometimes he gets his applause wherever he can.

Maybe the scholar and mythologist, Joseph Campbell, was right when he told us that heroes are chosen in some doctrine of naturalism, some random, before-we-were-born selection process. And we simply go along for the ride either as a participant, an observer, a fan, or an everyman.

This could be said of Christopher Reeve's willingness to go public with his plight, and of Dale Earnhardt accelerating into a turn at 230 mph in hopes of passing one more car. It could be said of Mantle, who played nearly his entire career injured. Every hero pays a price for the privilege, every man a price for his life.

According to Campbell's mythic archetype, the responsibility of heroes is to return to their "tribe" and share the knowledge gleaned on their Journey. My dad never recovered from cancer to tell me what it is like to have one's body devoured by metastasizing cells. Yet his struggle was played out for all of us to see—in his jaundiced-eyes and in his immutable will.

And the great Mick, who died from a hereditary disease and complications from alcoholism, was never able to return to the world from which he came and which adored him so. Like most men who give us feats of greatness before they develop feet of clay, his legend is larger than his life.

Carl Jung wrote,

> "The hero is a hero just because he sees resistance to the forbidden goal in all of life's difficulties and yet fights that resistance with the whole hearted yearning that strives towards the treasure hard to attain, and perhaps unattainable—a yearning that paralyses and kills the ordinary man."

On the baseball diamond, Mickey Mantle was a hero. Off it he was an ordinary man. And it killed him.

I wonder if my dad felt a hero's call. I never had the chance to ask him. On the morning that he died, he called each of us kids into his bed where he lay dying and said goodbye with dignity and prowess, unvanquished to the end. Propped up on three pillows, a little trickle of blood oozing out of the side of his smiling mouth, a hug, a kiss, and a strained voice asking us to take care of each other, as if he were sending us off to summer camp, a sleeping bag in one hand, a note on how to live a good life in the other. And then he was gone.

Tell me. Is there no difference between batting .325 for ten seasons in a row and raising seven kids on $1,400 a month? Does it matter which is greater: to be revered by a few or admired by millions? We need heroes in our lives, although I'm not so sure we know who they are anymore.

Roberto Clemente, arguably the best all-around baseball player of the modern era, is a hero not for his 3,000 hits or his seven Gold Glove Awards. No, I think of Clemente dying in a plane crash on the way to Nicaragua to help victims of a massive earthquake. For *that*, he was heroic. On the baseball field, he was a very talented athlete. We must not confuse the two.

I wonder if it would have made a difference if my dad had died suddenly and violently, without the eighteen months of gradual and relentless decline. Would he seem more of a hero and less a victim? Would my faith and understanding in his passing be any different if God had simply reached down with His hand and plucked him cleanly from this earth, sparing him the ultimate human embarrassment— bodily impression of a deity's ambivalence?

Sometimes we make our own decisions, sometimes they are made for us. And sometimes the two run together. Some athletes retire at the top of their game so as to never allow the public to witness their inevitable decline. Others, like my dad, have no choice, forced out by injury or illness.

On occasion I try to tell my own son what his grandpa would have been like, how cool it would have been for the three of us to surf together. Most of the time I can't finish the conversation; too much past bubbling up like liquid earth from the core—hot, unstoppable, necessary. One day, when the moment was right, I told my son that my dad would have really liked him, that he might have become a hero to my father. Nine years old, he turned to me and held my shoulders between his little hands, just like I was supposed to hold his, and said, "Yeah but Dad, I bet you were kinda like his hero too."

Eighteen years on the road, chasing that thin, white fog line up and down the Pacific Coast Highway, chasing chalk lines hastily laid out on the decomposed granite dirt of a high school track, the black tile on the bottom of the pool printed forever on the top of my brain—it was time for me to leave the world of professional athletics.

A little better than average, I may have raced as though each day was irreplaceable. But for more years than I care to recount, the sun had set on that day, and I was losing to kids half my age. I was nobody's athletic hero anymore.

But there was a time, on the front nine of my career, when I impressed enough to earn that cultural label. Once, I was leading a triathlon that lasted nearly nine hours. With half a mile left to run and two young hotshots breathing down my neck, I had to piss so bad it was killing me. To stop, even to slow down, would cause me to lose the race. Knowing that a precise emotion requires precise action, I reached down, pulled my shorts to the side, relaxed the appropriate muscles as best I could, and let her fly. The finish line in sight, the crowd cheering, two young speedsters on my heels, urine flying, women pointing, people staring, old men wondering, kids laughing, I thought: fuck 'em all. I crossed the line first and began looking for a cup of water to rinse with.

As I walked away, proud as a damn peacock, an official-looking man approached me and asked, "Mr. Tinley?" I expected he was going to disqualify me and wreck the whole day. He simply stuck his hand out to shake mine, not worried that my fingers were wet with sweat and pee.

"I saw you dig deep," he said. "Really deep. Such resiliency. Almost a vet." Then he walked away, leaving me to wonder at the meaning of his words.

What had I survived? What was I almost a veteran of? A sport? A damn game?

I remembered that day not long ago and wished more than anything that my dad could have been there. Not to see me win, not to see someone call me a hero, but to see me answer a call and follow that path, an exploding rebel soul on a journey of its own and fate's making, regardless of the price. I imagined him seeing himself in me, a reflection made clear with the hand's swipe at a foggy mirror.

If I've learned anything about life, then I must know a little about dying. All I wanted was for my dad to know that I tried. I really tried. And when I think of my son trying, really trying to make me feel better about the death of *my own* dad, I know that he will be a hero to someone, as he already is to me.

We are defined by those ahead and behind and all around us. There can be no other way.

Prescript: I've known Nico Marcolongo for many years. He is a veteran of the Iraq conflict who served fourteen years as a U.S. Marine Officer. After the conclusion of his military service in February 2008, Nico joined the Challenged Athletes Foundation (CAF) where he leads the CAF Operation Rebound program for injured veterans and first responders. Nico co-founded a weekly surf clinic that is now an established form of therapy for injured veterans. But before he did all that, Nico had to rehabilitate himself after a period spent as an active-duty soldier in a theater of war. Within counseling circles, the concept of PTSD is relatively new. In WWII and the Korean War, according to the U.S. government 2% of the returning soldiers suffered long term effects from involvement in these conflicts. But that seems an unreliable data point. It was not until 1980 that the US government created a name and a rubric for this movable malady. The government has also concluded that 5% of Vietnam War vets have been diagnosed, 14% of Persian Gulf War vets, and 15% of subsequent Iraq and Afghanistan conflict soldiers have, at some level, faced the vagarious and debilitating effects of those wars. If we consider that early versions of PTSD were reduced to the term "shell shock" during WWI and pay attention to the rise in psychological trauma associated with subsequent 20th and 21st century wars, we must also suggest that an entire generation of returning veterans are faced with their own personal rehabilitation.

Semper-Free

ST: *Prior to your deployment abroad, were you ever aware of any personal feelings, habits, thoughts, or mannerisms that might signal the challenges you were going to face upon return?*

Nico: Not at all. While it's inherent among service members that there are risks of being wounded or killed, the mental health risk of war was not something that was generally discussed or pondered.

ST: *Was there a point when you'd "hit bottom" and were in serious trouble?*

Nico: About seven months into an eight month Iraq deployment I experienced my first episode of major depression. I had no idea what hit me. I had never experienced anything like it previously. It was the worst torment I had ever endured. The anxiety felt like I was being pierced by thousands of needles. I felt a need to crawl out of my own skin. The depression weighed me down like a ton of bricks, I had to be very deliberate just to get out of bed. The pain was ceaseless and excruciating yet, physically, I was fine. It was hard to comprehend what was happening, why I was experiencing such debilitation and when and how it would end. It was something for which I was not prepared. These feelings lasted for about six months. A big factor was identifying the right medication in the right dosage.

ST: Can you describe some of the early feelings and experiences that you had when you came back from the war and realized you might be facing psychological challenges?

Nico: I did not realize until I was out of a war zone that I had PTSD. Hearing helicopter rotors as they flew overhead, loud noises, trash piles on the side of the road, etc. all elicited a physiological response of hyper-awareness and intrusive thoughts. I knew then that depression was a symptom of PTSD.

ST: Was there ever a plan or strategy to help with your PTSD? Were there others involved with that plan?

Nico: Yes, though it developed and evolved over time. The first thing was to find the right med. This was trial and error. It took about three months to get the right medication and dosage. After that, it was building an extended support community (family, friends, mental health professionals, fellow veterans).

ST: Describe what was going through your mind as you started to map out the rehab.

Nico: It was an unknown entity for me. It was my first experience with the military, or any for that matter, mental health system. With that, I knew that I needed help, so I overcame any reluctance to seek it. I knew that in my present condition at that time, I would not be able to function as a Marine Leader or more generally, as a husband and father. My goal was to be "combat effective" again. So, I began the process of meeting with physiatrists, counselors, and ensuring that I was doing things that aided in my healing such as eating right, getting sufficient sleep, exercising and focusing on getting better.

ST: Can you discuss the issues that you faced as you did "the work" to find your way back to emotional health?

Nico: The first thing was recognizing that I needed to get help. Next was understanding that there was something that I could do to get better, though initially it did not feel that way. I had to separate what I felt from what I knew. As the meds began to work and the deep fog of depression lifted, I felt relaxed but exhausted, as if my body had been through an arduous and stressful situation for an extended period. Giving myself time to recover, giving myself some grace, was a new experience for me but something that I knew that I needed to do if I was going to allow my body to heal.

ST: What were some of the highs and lows of your rehabilitation?

Nico: High points were discovering that I was not alone in what I was going through. Finding other veterans who had a similar experience and using my experience to help others. Lows were realizing that I was susceptible to such an injury, it was quite humbling. However, over time, I've come to accept it as a sacrifice of my service.

ST: Were there moments of clarity or frustration as you found your way back to normalcy?

Nico: Yes and no. Let me think about that.

ST: What were some of the key things that enable your recovery? Were they people? Meds? Counseling? Group discussion?

Nico: In addition to medication for depression and anxiety, I put an ad in the paper for a Marine Officer support group. My thought that other officers would be comfortable speaking with their peers about what they were experiencing. After a couple of months of not hearing from anyone, I got an email from a Marine spouse. She stated that her husband wasn't an officer but was struggling after coming back from Iraq. I said, "O.K., I'll meet with him." It turned out that we served in the same area of operations. Eventually, the support group grew and was led by Vietnam Veterans. I also had counseling. While it was helpful, the meds and being with fellow veterans, knowing that I was not alone in what I was going through, was most helpful.

ST: Was there an "a ha" moment when you knew you were going to be all right?

Nico: When the anxiety lifted followed by the depression, I knew that I was coming out of the woods. It took about six months. However, I also knew I had additional work to do. I still found myself hyper-aware and feeling guarded against potential threats. With that, with the cloud of depression lifted, I became more aware of potential PTSD triggers which allowed me to more deliberately confront them and more readily deal with their impacts in a constructive manner.

ST: Are there thoughts, feelings, or experiences that you've taken from the war and are able to hold onto and serve you in a positive light now?

Nico: Yes, definitely. I believe I'm more in-tune and to a larger degree empathetic with others who may be struggling with an injury or other challenges. This has suited me well in my current job as the CAF Operation Rebound program lead and more generally in relating with others. With that, it's also helped me to develop a more authentic self which, in turn, has allowed me to become more introspective. With authenticity comes more accountability, both self-accountability and holding others to account. Being authentic helps to break down facades and get to the heart of a matter.

ST: Given the option to choose a different past, perhaps not in the military, would you have gone in a different direction?

Nico: Joining the Marine Corps and becoming a Marine Officer was one of the best decisions that I ever made. I would not have changed that. While my PTSD was a result of my service, being a Marine and gaining the skills, resolve, and leadership that I developed in the Corps far outweighed the adversities of my injury.

SECTION 4:

REHAB OF LIFE TRANSITION AND CHANGE

Introduction

The 60s mega-band, The Doors, lost its lead singer, Jim Morrison to an overdose of drugs and alcohol in 1971, partially because he refused to embrace the idea of rehab. Interesting, for a self-styled, "warrior poet" to ignore concepts becoming of his personal ideology connected to "healing spirits." Other famous and infamous public musical figures (Brian Jones, Jimi Hendrix, Janis Joplin, Kurt Cobain, Courtney Love, et al.) who have either suffered or died at the hands of chemical abuse or disease represent the ideals of abuse-to-rehab in an awkward and incomplete light. Were their lifestyle/pathologies the symptoms or the symbols of a culture that embraced recreational drugs for all the wrong (or right?) reasons? Perhaps we do not understand what rehab is and is not.

How can anyone ever predict how a change in life circumstances—whether medical, occupational, relational or ideological—will affect their lives?

My hunch is that it has a lot to do with flexibility and acceptance. With transitioning from one world into another.

There are periods in a person's life that require adaptation and the ability to reframe one's place in the world. That new place might be living in a war-free environment, a love-free environment, no smoking on planes, no long hair, no shoes, no shirt, no service.

And so the kinds of rehab-in-transition can range from cancerous, soul-sucking bone pain, lit by a single, swaying, sixty-watt bulb in your tenement basement as you curse God for your fate, to a month-long stay in a posh, hillside, mocktail-serving Malibu "facility," that caters to the victims of such first-world maladies as sex addiction and gambling concerns. The similarities might surprise you; carryovers reminding us that rain falls on the just and the unjust. The common denominator is that things change.

And to survive, you must change.

It is estimated in their lifetime, nearly 23% of the adult population in the U.S. will enter some form of substance or behavioral-reform rehab program. But what about the simple but complicated effects of a child going off to college and leaving the parents empty-nested? What about the assassination of a public figure? A pandemic? A food shortage? The death of a loved one? Amputation? Blindness? An acne breakout on your first date? Bankruptcy? Losing relevancy? Gaining weight?

And what about the healing from living through those multiplicities of war? Not just bullets flying from nation states who ain't playing nice but the wars of arguments over property lines and safe-at-first-base and who had more than their share on the bar-bill? Do these momentary transitions and challenges and their effects on your place in life require that you make that 1-800 CALL to "someone who will be there to help?"

Perhaps rehabilitation is the most egalitarian part of human suffering. And what is rehabilitation other than adapting to change?

Prescript: In looking at life's transitions and challenges, and the resiliency required to return to a pain-free life, it dawned on me that a significant common denominator was both loss of love and the strength found in negotiating that loss. In failed relationships, it might be easy to see this paradox. But in other cases of injury, illness, or occupational loss, for example, it is less obvious. Loss of youth is loss of love by others who love us for being young. Returning veterans will speak of love for their fellow soldiers. COVID-19 challenged us to find new ways of loving someone online. Before that, the HIV crisis of the early 90s redefined how "protected" one needed to be before engaging in sexual if not loving relationships. A child leaving home doesn't mean you love that child any more or less, it just means that the way you love them has changed. As I claim, I know little really, about what love is. But as I have pondered these liniments of rehabilitation on some deeper level, the notion of love lost, love gained, and just "Godammit, why can't I get over them" still rearing their head in my heart. The essay below is my attempt to understand love and the effects of its loss. When I finished it, I had more questions than answers. But I felt that in my handful of pages, I'd come closer to some understanding. And I appreciate more and forever the people I feel have loved me despite my many faults.

Another Four-Letter Word: An Unprofessional Look at Love and Its Failings

> *"All the good things that had belonged to her vanished with her love."*
>
> —From the Greek myth, *Eros and Psyche*

> *"This is how I would die into the love I have for you: as pieces of cloud dissolve into sunlight."*
>
> —Rumi, *Sufi mystic and poet*

Sandra Skirts knew what she was doing. She had perfected the art of the pencil-drop-and-roll to such a degree that it would find its intended place below my fifth-grade desk on a regular basis. I'd reach down to pick it up, the corner of my eye catching her uncross those brown ankles, the patent leather saddle shoes swaying like a metronome.

"Is this yours?" I'd ask in some pre-pubescent game and her brown saucer eyes would have me all the way until sixth period English. Damn, she was good.

I drove by the house that Sandra grew up in last week. There was foil on the windows and in the driveway sat the same '72 Country Squire Wagon that her father had bought new for "just under three big ones."

"Look at the wood veneer, son," he boasted. "Now, that's real laminate, my boy ... real wooden plastics."

That was right before Sandra, and I went to the junior prom and eighteen months before her dad died of Hodgkin's. I missed the funeral because I was in Israel pretending to grow tomatoes in a Kibbutz. I'm not Jewish but like many of the unholy acts of our past, it sounded like a good idea at the time. I don't think Sandra ever forgave me for missing her father's funeral. We'd been split up for almost six months by then and even though she was smarter than me, I was away at college, and she had been at home taking care of her dad and studying to be a library technician. I'm not sure what went wrong, really. But that's a poor interpretation of a powerful past.

I know exactly what happened.

Sandra and I used to lie on our backs in the park after school and imagine shapes in the clouds. One Friday in early spring, the same week her father had claimed he was in "re-commission" from cancer, and we had seen our picture sitting together at lunch in the school yearbook, a huge cumulonimbus floated by. I said it looked like a giant square-rigger beating to weather in an ancient sea. She said it looked like a toaster oven. I was unafraid of inconsequential consequence. She was sweet and loved small dogs more than small people. Sandra Skirts was growing old too young. She was Candide to my Pangloss.

And since her father claimed he had "never skirted an issue in his life" he would survive and give her away at the altar. But a lot of things ended that spring Friday, including me and Sandra. The clouds went dark, and we walked home in the rain, glad for the sound of thunder to interrupt our darker thoughts.

Years later when I was back in town for a weekend, we spent our one and only evening together. My grand square-rigged ship was now a cargo vessel, and her toaster oven was a lovely new kitchen remodeled with money left over from life insurance. There was never a chance for any sad wisdom in compromise. It was a thing of youth but with emotionally mortal stakes.

=====

It's been said by many wistful thinkers that love is the opening of possibilities, that it can set you free and send your heart soaring. But like a hubris-ridden athlete before a big game or a criminal blurting his mea culpa as he stands in judgment, the philosophers of love are often driven to their creative edges while living on their own emotional cusps; the beginning and ending of anything always conjuring grand ideas, joy and pathos. The miserable, the mundane and the serial monogamous, they rarely say much that we remember. Make no mistake, there are many artists who seek and find their pathos, purposely sabotage relationships, and will generally fuck up their love-lives for the sake of a few good paragraphs, a significant verse or a lasting canvas.

I am not sure if my art is that misanthropically refined. More so it feels like my heart is like a piñata—it needs to get beat with a stick to find out what's really inside. Or maybe there is just enough inherent danger in failed love to even out the beauty and joy when a real romantic relationship is really happening.

This is the fault of love or perhaps more specifically, the ambiguity of love.

We are socially inscribed to mistake lust for love, innately wired to confuse true admiration for unconditional devotion, and to fear falling in love for fear of the pain of falling out of love. And from back when Aphrodite ordered her son, Eros to play that fateful trick on Psyche, until the present-day ethos of Reality TV-consciousness, games of heartfelt-consequence continue to be played while we remain confused about love and its role(s) in our world.

Take the institution of marriage. The myth is that vows and promises are to be upheld regardless. The truth is that people don't always evolve in the same direction let alone make the effort to weave enough similar threads to sustain the eventual strain.

I don't know if too many people stay married for the wrong reasons or if too many people get divorced for what they think are the right reasons. Like the poet said, "the longer we were married, the closer we grew apart."

Since 5th grade, I've only been married once and in romantic love 3.25 times; two blondes and 1 ¼ brunettes, though the fraction lady had a seasonally dependent hair shade. I'm hardly qualified to make any claims on the subject. But I remember the beginnings and the endings. And I remember most of the middles.

One of the problems in discussing love is that every participant in the conversation not only has their own filter, radar, and protective heat shield on but is in a different current state of emotion. How can you agree that the sky is blue when some cultures don't have a word for that shade and others are simply color blind? Can you imagine what it would be like if other social institutions were so contextual? Imagine walking into church and having the preacher tell you that he'd had a change of heart about Jesus Christ as savior because he'd cut his palms with a nail by accident and then had been robbed by a Hispanic kid named Jesus? People seem to relate to love more based on how it let them down than how it propped them up. This is not to empower cynicism. More so it may reflect the temporal aspects of a relationship as we remember the pain of a breakup *after* the joy of falling in love.

Shakespeare realized this best when opting to approach love through tragic comedy. By writing a drama that makes us both laugh and cry in the same scene he was able to re-create exactly what love does—it makes us *feel*. And to feel things powerfully is perhaps the best way to remind ourselves that we are, after all, alive. And to combat existential angst by embracing the outrageous fortunes of living is not so essential as it is basic survival. This might explain why some desire to be in love and then subconsciously sabotage the relationship. It's like the soldier who re-enlists after returning from the theater of battle—war is hell but at least you feel more alive than sitting on your parent's coach in Duluth with a quart of Jack Daniels watching Ricky Lake re-runs.

Shakespeare also has this whole thing about forbidden love figured out. Whether considering the hilarity and joy that ends A *Midsummer Night's Dream* or the deep despair of *Romeo and Juliet*, it's what forbidden love *signals* that resonate with us, not the love itself. Of course, we all pine for the happy ending but must realize that forbidden love is love without the shackles of social or morally inscribed pressures. Both in myth and in practicality, it represents our species' desire to be with who we want to be with; to love *autotelically* or only for the sake of itself.

Still, forbidden love is much less sustainable than when those social and moral support systems get a couple through the tough times.

This is not to argue for multiple partners or less commitment to the notion of allowing love to grow and develop over time. Not at all. But in a time when love— like other areas of "humanness" that were previously considered unassailable—- we find the truest of true things mediated and manipulated to such an extent that deciding if we really *do love* someone now requires a great degree of personal insight and honesty.

Maybe it's harder to really like someone than to fall in love with them.

While saying "I love you" on a regular basis is a learned pattern that would please any constructivist, I'm not sure that there hasn't been a cost to verbalizing those three words when we don't mean it. Given a choice though, I'd vote for error on the side of supply, not demand.

And if you are in love with whom you are presently with, then consider yourself very lucky or very good or more likely, your partner is also very good and sort of lucky. Still the notion of "earning" love has some merit. It must be considered a privilege not a right. The notion of *free love*—rampant during the 1960s resistance to conservative values—often ceased to be free nine months *ipso facto*.

Of course, this is all contrary to the idea that real love is simple, easy, tangible and above all, obvious. But love is blind, right?

===

I believe in love at first sight. I believe in soulmates, and I believe that yes, love does conquer all. But I also believe that the purposeful and contiguous act of being in love is analogous to that circus game of *whack-a-mole* where lots of players try and beat down the mole with a club and win the prize. It takes a variety of skills to gain quickness, patience, observant eyes, and willingness to go the distance. Love is the mole that is destined to win because he cannot lose. He will forever rear his head regardless of how bad we beat him. The Mole, Love, knows that the club we wield is as soft or as hard as our willingness to accept a cheaper imitation of one of the last true currencies of value—unconditional love between humans.

Love is perhaps best defined by what it is not. It is not mediocre or malevolent, passionless or purposeful, stoic or stagnant. It does not ask for nor give advice. Love does not go lightly into any good night, nor will it shine forever unless mutually re-powered. And it does not mean *never having to say you're sorry.*

Love does not stand on the edge of reason and will not jump unless pushed from behind. Some days it can be what two or more people agree it is for the moment. But how many relationships are sustainable when found on an early and blurry agreement to agree? As French, Cuban/Spanish writer, Anaïs Nin suggest, "Love never dies a natural death. It dies because we don't know how to replenish its source."

And when it fails, the world can implode. Fewer are the failed relationships that are catalyzed by one party than the couple who mutually and equally look at each other and decide, "This isn't going anywhere. Why don't we just end this?" More so, failed love is for one party, either mildly traumatic or a psychic catastrophe. It doesn't seem fair to fault anyone for not loving someone anymore, but certainly the timing and touch of a breakup can have a big effect on the rehabilitation of the uh ... victim. I remember reading about "Dear John" letters that found their way into the hands of soldiers fighting in theaters of war abroad and wondering what's worse? Dogging bullets or knowing that your sweetheart would be dating some peacenik that got out of the draft on a trumped up 4F.

One of my friends who is a bit of an intellectual romantic (oxymoron?) told me that "Love is transmutable, therefore evolving." His claim took me a while to digest but, in the end, I decided he only meant that you could never put your finger on what love is and what it's not. When I asked him, "What's harder: falling in love or falling out of love?", he just mumbled Homer Simpson-like, "Hmmm, depends ... really depends."

Quite often, love *is* an inner marker of an outward state. It can be a map or a myth, a place or a feeling of placeless-ness. It can be tall ships *and* kitchen appliances so long as they move in sync, downwind or into the eye of the storms. Once love gets into your marrow, it may be suppressed, even ignored. But you cannot fully kill that what which has owned you. It goes into some deep recess of your brain until after your divorce is final, and you find out on Facebook that your college sweetheart is now single …

Love is strange that way.

Only it can break your heart.

═══

I have no desire to seek out Sandra Skirts if even to test my theory of deep compartmentalization. She is married, I've heard, lives far away on a farm with kids and dogs and books and farming things. But there is a romantic that lurks in all of us and sometimes he resides just below the surface, other times in those dark crevices. We want to remember young love because we've had a chance to erase the pain of breaking up, to sugar coat it with sweet nostalgia and better times. But after that *first time*, our memories of love are subject to a kind of emotional McCarthyism, an unnatural force that unfairly lumps all love together and catalyzes such totalizing claims as, "Well, if it was meant to be, it would've been."

Bullshit on that, I say. Too many factors in our postmodern world affect our life-chances at finding a mate who we actually have love-ish feelings for. Lots of us construct our defenses around avoiding failure instead of achieving success. We can dance around each other like junk yard dogs in the dust or Disney characters on the ballroom floor. But love should never be played like a zero-sum game. People get hurt with love.

Love sucks.

Yeah, but love is life.

Still, love should never be regrettable.

I should've gone to the funeral.

═══

I don't wish that love would've been easier in my life by counting love on one hand minus 1.75 fingers. Forget whether it's paternal, maternal, romantic or otherwise; love still remains, for most of us, an interpretable act that confounds, confuses, and leaves us wondering whether to take her home or pour him into a taxi and think "Whew, that was close. I actually liked that one." But how can we know love if we don't let it know us? And new-agey as it sounds, how can we let love know us if we can hardly recognize what he/she/it stands for?

My friend Jimmy Hunter knows love well. It has taken him 58 years, four marriages, three divorces, two near-death accidents, the passing of one of his parents, the rearing of four children, three of which he thinks he fathered, and the rise and fall and rise of a multiplicity of ideologies to realize that no one can really *know* love. Jimmy just likes people.

And that's how he has come to know what love means.

But he also likes sex which—he has come to realize—can be the undoing of love. The separation of love and sexual relations should be easy to understand. The pragmatist knows that one has understandably contextual connections though each situation in and of itself is a slippery slope. One is an act, the other acted upon for reasons that are often dangerously close to, and interfaced with, love.

But not to adhere too closely to my Roman Catholic roots, excuse me if I remind our readers that good stories (and by extension, exciting endings) are often based on rising tension and then release. Take away tension and release and you dull not only the story but erase the human species, if you follow the orgiastic reference. Love, sex, and good narratives allow a resonant tale to slowly gather steam, create conflict, increase the tension and then resolve the issue, all the while in an effort to make sense of the episode in what the French labeled the dénouement, the resolution of all conflict and catharsis.

That's where the post-coitus cigarette must've been lit. That's where love-gone-away and rehab begin.

While that might be a proper directive for the author to craft on the page, it's something else altogether to live out in a long-term relationship where the word *love*, in its overuse, has come mean both feelings for wine, grandchildren, and a new season of that throne game. Certainly, the word, in its pervasive appropriation by those-that-mean-well-but-maybe-not, has been used-to-death. While Johnny Cash called it a "burning thing" and Bob Dylan countered with the claim that "love is just a four-letter word," popular culture's embroidery of the term has only served to highlight what authenticity is left in the meaning and action behind the symbolic interpretation.

Real love is like rain, hard in sound, soft to the touch. Break ups are just hard.

====

Some days I think I wish I wanted to be falling in love. I want to be all goo-goo and ga-ga like in the other first days when I was barely legal, just married or barely just old enough to get shot with my own gun. I want to know that I am human because love and its resultant plethora of emotions remind me so. I want to wake up, smell the coffee and think that is the odor of love. But as *en vino veritas* I do know that there is truth in wine, love, and in well-prepared coffee.

Still, there are always barriers to love. Blame it on the tequila or that other big worm that tempted Eve in the Garden. Blame it on the kids, the dog, the creditors or the clouds. Blame it on your spouse.

Blame it on your fear of leaving or finding a spouse.

But don't blame it on love itself. At least one thing left must remain unvanquished.

And perhaps only love or the pain of its demise can play that role well enough.

Prescript: The following piece of fiction was based on several friends of mine who came back from the Vietnam and Gulf Wars. They had changed. Their choices and behavior during extended rehabilitation is juxtaposed here against the surf heroes of my youth, the men and women who were good enough or lucky enough to avoid war, who made my boards, who surfed better than anyone on the block. Surfing, if nothing else, represents eternal youth, freedom, and expression. Just the opposite of militarism. But a lot of surfers went to Vietnam and the Middle East to serve and fight. And I always wondered how their chosen lifestyle and sport choices before and after deployment affected their return and rehabilitation. Perhaps there is some truth to how big wave surfers make good soldiers. Consider their fearlessness and focus. I wonder if it's true that NASA, when looking for individuals to enter the original Mercury 7 program, interviewed big wave surfers. The intent in this story was to avoid the pitfalls of projected guilt surrounding those who served and those who stayed home and surfed. I wanted to let a singular character's mind speak for a generation who were faced with unpopular wars. And who returned home changed. Or who had used the dreams and metaphors of surfing to explain the nightmares and analogs of war. I missed the Vietnam War draft by less than six months. Maybe 18 if I was feeling lucky. My draft number was 13. In January of 2025, my wife and I spent a few weeks in the Republic of Vietnam. We climbed through the Cu Chi tunnels outside Ho Chi Hinh City and it scared the fuck out of us. I tried to surf small, hapless surf at China Beach outside Danang, and the local lifeguard told me that it was forbidden due to the danger of dying.

Only When It's Necessary

In the shaping cellar, the single swinging light bulb no longer interrogates my past. In those days after my first tour, I was still a solitary figure more opt to bend a little than be swayed. Maybe I wasn't that curious about what war meant. I know that I went there, and people died, and I didn't. The entire post-war decade might've been a hangover for some. But I was mowing off something else.

My parents left me this place and everything in it. After a stint in a Huntington surf ghetto, I came east in '75. Not sure why. Something about re-rooting my core.

Lots of people in Hastings, Nebraska have converted bomb shelters; concrete holes in the middle of the yard justified by Weather Channel hyperbole and the quadrennial twister. How they've converted them nearly defines the owners. Some families have bible study groups on *Revelations*. Some guys have CB radios. Others have elaborate crack labs with video surveillance. Mine ended up as a surfboard shaping room because I used it as bait; an earthen lair requiring me to crawl back into a hole in the ground from which something new and beautiful might emerge.

The guy at the VA said I was trading one problem for another. I said I could live with the second problem but not the first. He wrote that down. I told him that I've managed to reshape the blanks into smaller and smaller problems, my Skil 100 a replacement for a thin paring knife aimed at my left ear.

When I came back in-country I was an off-the-rack guy. Now I realize that a good hand shape is like a good war—there is a perfect period for it to make a positive difference in a negative world. Before and after, it's just a bad idea or something grown into a horrible taste. I don't sell the boards I shape down there. Not a lot of core surfers in Hastings. So, they're stacked and ready for something of tectonic proportions to happen, a 100-year flood and all my neighbors are floating down a river of Kool-Aid on an unglassed 6' 6" piece of foam.

In a war, soldiers are restocked with something younger and fresher. The aging is violent. You don't breathe in war, you gulp. No one pauses to watch resin drip down the rail. And then you go home and close the curtains. Yeah, I don't mind it down there in the shaping cellar now. My visits are sometimes ponderous and sometimes like relatives and vital ghosts—they visit but I don't let them stay long. I consider the slender shapes, their gracious ends and rails flat against the old teak racks. Some days I imagine them as premature infants in a hospital window. Other times, they appear as sleek, shrink-wrapped body bags lying in slimming black atop the hard tarmac; maybe Tan Son Nhat or Baghdad International. The both of them waiting for a ride home—one cooking, the other cooked. I talk to them.

"We'll meet again, Little Brother. Stop by if you're ever in Hastings, NE. I'll make you a 5' 5" fish or if you live long enough, a gentleman's thruster or a precocious wall hanger made for conditions that wake you up at night."

On other nights like tonight, when I'm having friends over and have to go down there to grab a bottle of wine or to do some light finish sanding, I don't even turn on the light. I just reach for the high shelves where the good stuff is kept ... 220 grit paper labels. I feel just a bit closer to Jesus that way, knowing how, in the one story the man of sorrows turned the water into the good shit.

I told the new doc at the VA about that. He didn't write it down.

One time he tried to speak in surf tongues—*dude* and *gnarly* and *out the back*. I'm not talking about Jesus but the guy at the VA. He has a beard too. Grew it well before the plaid Malloy phenomenon. He said, "Son, don't go opening up a second front on yourself. You're safe in the World now."

I said "You mean the new war or the new world because the second front has always been when you freshly walk back into your stale home—that two-bedroom, two bath theater of ops with wall-to-wall memories of someone you don't know anymore. And he doesn't know you. You circle each other like sumo wrestlers, eyes fixed, mind fixed, neurons firing, unfriendly fire, a fire engine screams past but you don't live in the past. No room in the garage for even two sawhorses and standard seven-foot blanks. No one is asking you to take modern day tour of the Cu Chi tunnels outside of Saigon.

"You can still be that same kid from down the block," he said.

"The same as what?" I kept on this doc with lots of letters after his name but no fucking common sense. "Who should I be, Doc? The six-year-old who slept with his kitten on the pillow," I asked him, "or the fourteen-year-old who tied a bell to the cat's tail that drove him crazy and later, taught the cat to do aerials above the bathtub?

"Hey Doc, you still taking surf vacations to Typhoon Lagoon at Disney World?"

===

Billy and his wife are coming tonight. At least he said that they would. We don't hold each other responsible for social graces. I met Billy in the psych ward at Walter Reed in the summer of '73. We planned a trip to La Libertad figuring too many people would be afraid of the war down that way. Petty little pissing match between juntas. Great right hand cobbled points. Billy was diagnosed with neurotic paranoia. I had paranoid neuroses; both maladies indicting each other while all we wanted to do, was to make it go away in warm water and cold cervezas. Billy had loved the Hawaiians when he was on the North Shore in '68 and punched a kid from Florida in the mouth with a can of dog food from Kami's Market when the punk tried to steal a case of Top Ramen.

The war ends for a while when your buddy comes over and tells you how much they love the new stick. In the soldier, it's a forever rash that some people itch, and others scratch. You're back after your (fill in the blank here) tour and you've been de-briefed after being de-loused, defrocked and you tell yourself that you ain't deranged. That's just war talking. Trying to derail you from your long journey back to someplace that you won't recognize if you get there. Like going to Lazaro Cardenas for the first time after they built the damn. You just can't quite get your head around what was and now is.

That's why I hate Chinese pop-out boards. No room for negotiation. Dave Parmenter was right.

The war pundits used to say that evil should be written about the way it is or not at all. I don't know what that means. I read a lot of books when I came back. Could've taught college courses in Vietnam Lit or predicted the dearth of decent Gulf Lit. Some of it stuck to the brain-like sand on a dropped piece of fruit. Other shit was pinged off or burnt up as it tried to entire my atmosphere. This I know for sure. I think. As the world turns, so spins war. Blink and you'll miss a mass grave or two. Go on vacation and an entire uprising runs its due course like a one-day swell. The thing about wars is they end. And then they start over. The new swell wars hyped by the surf media are like little glass snowballs—shake up a few insurgents, check your photo-bonus contract, and then set it in the closet until next season.

Surfing too is different now, a bit better, a bit worse. But it's still there. Larry, my pal from Alpha Fiberglass, he was the one that got me the gig teaching high school history. He told me over a bottle of port that we've come to dealing with our wars in consonant sounds, euphonic letters that resonate and creep into the spaces that help us define dereliction of duty if not death. Larry says that the myth of murder has been collateralized by the machine and killing is traded on the open market, mediated in back rooms and war rooms and rigid-minded reactionaries as well as compartmentalizing, pseudo-hippy co-ops. I made Larry some abomination he refers to as a "fun shape." As opposed to what? A miserable-time-surfing shape?

Surfing has been reduced to smooth sounding words as well, he says. I tried that line on my school principal one time. I think he wanted to understand. But he hadn't earned it. He's an apocalyptic Gidget Guy—someone whose entire reference to riding waves and war has been shaped by popular culture.

Larry is a trip. I love his tight weave 4-ounce stuff.

In this grand commodification of war and surfing, we've lost site of the warrior surfer. It can be confusing for those who stay at home. Who can blame them? In modern war—the urban-jungle, remote control guerrilla type with manufactured enemies, divided supporters and IEDs made from children's shampoo-it gets pretty muddy. As wars get more obtuse, so goes the mind of the veteran surfer and surfing veteran. Or so went a lot of ours. There was so much clarity in Old School annihilation and power-drive bottom turns.

I hope Billy comes tonight. He's read Homer's work like six times and can quote Jack London on a dime. Said he didn't get Homer until the fifth. He says the thing about war parades and surf contests is that everybody on the sidelines thinks they know what is being celebrated and contested and then somebody always cleans up after them. Billy says that the modern Odysseus might be in a firefight in the Sudan on Friday and sitting down for dinner at his parents in Des Moines by Sunday. *Welcome home, son. Be sure to clean the dead skin under your fingernails before supper.* Very messy indeed.

Billy says pro surfers should be more gracious to locals. He says if someone like Slater or Parko were too aggressive in the lineup, it would be like Woods or Mickelson pushing their way through a crowded public par-3 course on a quiet Sunday morning. Billy was a recon guy. A full ghost for three tours. He goes back over there on vacation now. But he still just crawls around in the red mud looking for pieces of himself. We laugh about it now. It's a start. He says it's still Charlie's Point but for new reasons. Money buys you more shit than bullets I reckon.

I'm hoping that Little Jackie stops by tonight. She went to Iraq 1 in '90 as a systems operator; a buxom button pusher who has been trying to figure out cause and effect ever since. Gratuitous technology, I told her one night in the cellar as she watched me shape a 7' 6" pin tail for some guy up in Lincoln who grew up in La Jolla, did his basic at MCRD, and hasn't been in the Pacific since he was on leave at China Beach in May of '70. I told her about the machine shaping that all the big guys use now. She nodded and a kind of dark whimsy coated her eyes like a soapy film. I think we hugged and watched the light bulb pendulum. She's a good friend; solid as far as non-surfers go.

Yes sir, you'll have new friends when you come home from war or surfing the North Shore for the first time. More than you remember. Yep. They come, they go, unannounced with needs and gifts you can't possibly fill or use. They're a nuisance, really. And I didn't like having to argue with them. When I used to tell the other docs at the VA about them, they'd always lean in a little closer to me, like they were trying to smell the truth or something. "How big were those combers again, Son?" Then they'd write on their clipboard, and I could hear the point of the pen make that scratchy sound that echoed through the particle board and came out into the room. Little sounds that told my story filtered by ink and textbook-learning from another man who I wouldn't die for or even kill for. Even if I knew his story. Which I doubt he's about to tell me anytime soon.

I knew my war buddy's stories though. I knew their sister's middle name and their priest or rabbi's hometown. I heard their confessions, their vows, and their Bar Mitzvah blessing. I knew the size of their big wave guns and surf trunks and carburetor throat. I knew their blood type and wax preference. I saw everything in their eyes, swallowed through their eyes, behind them and in front of them.

The way they surfed. The way they fought.

And I let them see mine all the way past my core and into my past and my mother's past—the molten skeletons that hung and swayed outside our tents, aired by the fresh wind of all that is pure in war and surf trips. Which is only the love among soldiered surfers and not a damn thing else.

Yes sir, when you come home and know that you aren't going back, you start falling and there's not a soul that can catch you 'cept yourself. The only sure way to know it's final in this mercantile army of surf sales reps is to ensure that you're damaged goods. Return to sender. The modern army does a cost/benefit analysis on you. And then you're depreciated like a John Deere, or a uni-size Quicksilver trucker's hat made in China. You're alive but something's missing on the outside maybe and the inside for sure. Yes sir, this is a different war with good turtle-armor to keep you alive but damn if it's hard sewing toes and fingers and arms and what not back on the trunk. But parts are parts and you end up just like that line from Springsteen's *Jungle Land*—" *wounded*, not even dead."

Surfboards sold in Costco. The horror.

You start to look for answers but you ain't gonna' ever find them in the magazines or the for-profit surf report sites. Only in the water and the earth. The dirty sea contains dangerous levels of iron from the rust of dead fighting machinery and the blood of dead fighting men. You can't look down. The earth is Medusa and wants you to be sand to help dilute the minerals. So, you look up and hope to find something, a horizon that helps. Lot of guys found it too. But lots of guys end up like Lot's Wife.

======

Did you know that the human hand is the most dexterous piece of machinery ever produced by man or God? Nothing has ever been created that can function in more angles and degrees and points of articulation. Entire languages are spoken with the hand. And they only use a fraction of the shapes and forms imaginable and functional with the human hand. But if you take away just a piece, a little piece even, it changes the entire operation. Laws of physics, man. Think about an 18-wheel truck missing just one eighth of one tire. That thing won't even stay upright. Falls over like a child's top. I could shape a decent nose rider with a sharpened stone and my two hands. You could park yourself on the tip for days if I got the nose concave shaped just right.

Yes sir, I was in tip-top tight shape over there. And things were measured in degrees of tension. My tight gut and tight unit set against a loose objective or none at all. My tight biceps and tight platoon carrying out loose ops. Some guys had a tightness all the way into piano wire. High octave, G sharp territory. Guys who tried to stay in tune for their whole tour broke more than themselves trying to play any tune that wasn't discordant. Lotta surfers in the lineup are strung pretty tight these days. They don't surf as much as they snap their chips from one publishable position to the other.

I don't ever remember anything snapping when I came back, and it wasn't even a sense of unwinding the bands. It was more like you were just used to living with that degree of intermittent tension. You needed it, expected it, it held you, guided you. The tension defined you. But it didn't function in the water. The ocean pushed back until I submitted and let her take me. Rag dolled through two wave hold-downs and came up laughing because I came up loose.

But back on land when the tension wasn't there the world felt soggy, marsh-like with no spring. Each step was accentuated, and you had time to watch your foot enter the earth and it required more effort to pull it back out again. That was the hardest thing to get used to—walking back in the World.

I had sex-with-meaning with a nurse that I met at the Surf Theater in Huntington Beach in June of 1973. *Five Summer Stories Plus One* was playing. I wish I could remember her name. She had the most exotic ankles. One afternoon when we were at the Food Basket buying green onions for tomorrow's omelet, she told me that vets and surfers have great capacities, great piles of love to give and holes that need filling. But their way of trying to make the equilibrium well, equal, is foreign to the World. In the checkout line she said that like in soldiers, in surfers there is hidden tenderness to their rage and buried anger just below the surface of their kindness. In the parking lot she told me that the modern surfer's two new enemies are other surfers and the surfing industrial complex. I wondered if it has been that way for a long time and told her that the philosopher William James predicted this over a century ago. "War and adventure," I quoted from his *The Varieties of Religious Experiences*, "assuredly keep all those who engage in them from treating themselves too tenderly."

Lynnette and I stayed in bed well past breakfast on Tuesday. Was that LA or San Francisco? I wish I could remember her name.

Larry thinks that surfing now is different, like wars are different. One guy at the VA-smart doc told me that surfing, like war, is a social construct. It's like a book club or a group of guys getting together to play hoops on Sunday morning. He said it means that people actively choose their interactions between others as opposed to having them imposed upon them. I asked him what about getting drafted. He said that was a thing of the past; that war will now become a profession, a high-tech robotic thing fought over basic material resources like trees and water. And waves? I asked. "If it comes to that," he said. "If it comes to that."

He seemed to like that suggestion and left the room musing to himself, sounding like Homer Simpson, "Mmmm … coming to that."

My nurse with the ankles thought that modern war is like a B-List sponsored pro surfer—they require a bit of cosmetics to get in the door, a lot of PR to keep them noticed, and tend to fade from public view while they pine at their craft with great mediocrity. We were trading metaphors between body parts that day, so I said you mean Iraq 1 was like one of those Mexican standoffs with a wild *javelina* on an old desert road headed for Puerto? Neither side wanted each other there. Neither knew quite how it got to that point and neither man nor beast is willing to move an inch. I wish I could remember Lynette's name.

Things have changed so much since *this* war started. We're out of soldiers. Out of breath. Out of a lot of things. But not Gaza or Ukraine.

===

Once you have surfed perfect Punta Unnamed you don't ever really come back, do you? You checked that box and then looked for another to jump into. Something with high risk and higher reward. The best commodities traders I've seen were great guys to explore surf with, front line cats from Iraq 1 who thought Gorden Gekko was a pussy and Darwin's work was unfinished. "Who cares if greed is good or if the environment shapes our being?" they'd ask. "The importance is in controlling one's destiny."

These are *fish-or-cut bait* guys with seven figure incomes. For them, life ain't bad on account they won't let it be. They're *glad* for the malaria at Nias and think Tavarua is under-developed.

The first month I was back wasn't so bad. It was sort of like a reverse honeymoon. But after I started sleeping in the closet, I knew there was work to do. It wasn't just the war but every part of my life that I had written in ellipses wanted to be filled in. The kid I'd found hanging in his own closet, the years I'd spent on the road running down a dream, the missed dinners, the vomited mistakes, the people I'd hurt and the ones who'd cut me, the in-laws, bylaws, maydays, highways and bad days all jumped out of the bibliography of my life and demanded real foot notes. It was a good thing. The story took ten years and thousands of pages to tell. But among many things, telling it taught me that there are only two things worse than dying. One is only a part of you dying and the other I can't remember. But it was bad.

REHAB … COLLECTED STORIES AND ESSAYS ON RESOLUTION, RESILIENCY, AND RETURN

The closer I get to the basic form of a shape, the clearer it becomes that there is no real vocabulary for any surf or war story except a straightforward telling. Some days I exist precisely nowhere, the compass of my *surform* looking for true north. I have but one toe in desire and the other in intuition. I hear voices emanating from thin dark eyes buried beneath thinner straw lids and rolls of light cloth wrapping round brown eyes. They say, "There it is."

There it is.

In my lighter moments I realized that surfing, just like in Vietnam, will keep coming, year after year, decade after decade. I asked Larry if he thought that after every Vietnam vet and 60s surfing hero were dead there wouldn't be anyone to tell of the countless dead in the counting years to come or perfect empty Rincon in '53. He always and already that surfers and soldiers will die and come back to us in the stories of the survivors. The living though they go on living.

Larry is sometimes too smart for my own good. He has crow's feet around his eyes; they are quote marks for all the good things he's told.

If he wasn't working as a school counselor, he would make a great glasser or maybe a shrink. I like Larry. We'll drink the top shelf stuff tonight. And then I'm going to show him the rhino chaser. He'll see that I left Vietnam only to think far into the East, trading one for another, a Far for a Middle. He'll see that I know war and three wave hold downs.

He and I both know that old warriors will always have to rise up through the cracks like weeds on a forgotten sidewalk, finding the one patch of nutrient dirt to sustain themselves in the sun while the world walks over them. There may be a few of the oddly unvanquished, the dark greenies who'll grow roots big enough to split the deafening concrete casement around them. Or maybe they're just sane enough to know that concrete and a good reef are just rocks and sand anyway.

Most of the vets are left to the mercy of the wind and rain until they can find some womb of the world with a few friends around who speak the language. Yeah, under the earth, man-built to save himself from himself. Shaping cellars. Dust to dust. Foam to foam.

And there we'll wait. Until the next big one. It'll make '58, '69, and '83 look like Newport Dunes on a hot August night. You see, it just isn't right to live under anybody's bad cloud. Especially your own.

"I gotta go Doc. I'll see you tonight."

Prescript: A lot of my friends are looking at cutting back on their workload if not retiring altogether. For some, it is a wondrous new chapter in their life journey. For others it is an unexpected and fearful shift in identity. The character profiled below, Tom Warren, is perhaps the most iconoclastic person I know. His various "projects" were prescient to the newfound challenges of hybrid-style occupations. I find Warren fascinating because he has never been in rehab yet has been rehabilitating himself for over sixty years. This profile of Warren is meant to call out the nuances and similarities of retirement and transition—a kind of rehabilitation in and of itself. Our post-COVID world offers us a plethora of work-condition options. But as all these baby boomers age up and out of the workforce, we wonder if they or the social world they help create are ready for it.

Good Work, if You Can Get It

> *"Man is not just in search of tensions per se, but in particular, in search of tasks whose completion might add meaning to his existence."*
>
> —Viktor Frankl, *Man's Search for Meaning*

Tom Warren works very, very hard. As an NCAA swimming star at USC, a successful real estate investor, and a business owner, you would expect him to be cut off from some carbon fiber-weave of industrial cloth. But Warren is a wood and steel guy, not Old School but indefinable in the prescient style of Steve Jobs or the Rolling Stones. To the casual observer, he is a ball of perpetual motion rolling as if dropped onto a practice billiards game that no one is really concerned about. But there is purpose in his movement, even if he is the only one who knows the rules of his game.

Warren knows something about work and physical culture that we do not. On the night after he won the 1979 Hawaiian Ironman Triathlon, he went out walking in the rain. No reason: it just seemed like something to do.

===

The lure of occupational stereotyping is a strong one. It's an easy trap in a liberal democratic political economy. What we do for our labor if not our primary remuneration must nearly define and stratify us. It's a safe and sane way to subvert the conversational work of getting to know someone. "Oh, you're an accountant! How ... *formulaic* your life must be," we might suggest. Or "Oh, you own real estate! It must have been nice to be born with money." And "Oh, you've competed in triathlons! Then you've done that race in Hawaii where they swim through lava. Do you strain your cottage cheese to reduce the fat content?"

Tom Warren is now in his mid-70s though he looks 10 or 15 years younger depending on the lighting and analogs lurking about the room. When he won the Ironman World Championship in 1979 and went on to finish in the top 3 in1980 and 1981, Warren would list his occupation as *saloonkeeper*. His saloon, *Tug's Tavern*, had been variously hailed in the press as, "a biker-bar dive", "a friendly local pub", and "the best place for late night munchies in Pacific Beach." While the descriptives were accurate enough, it was Warren's work to service the projected clientele that made the place profitable. I used to see Tom running on the Mission Beach Boardwalk around noon while I took my own lunch hour break from a decent but unsustainable position in the area. On occasion he would write notes to himself in the sand to remind him of a thought on his return route.

"How does he do it?" I'd ask myself, "How does one man so purposely dream, design, and create an occupation that allows him to swim, bike, and run by day and pour beer to his pals at night?"

Years later, after we become friends and training partners, I would ask Tom about this. And in his indefatigable response he would go on and on about how he'd never worked a day in his life. But he'd sure put a lot of effort into doing things that gave him pleasure and oh, by the way, paid the rent. Most people would just be winding you up with a comment like that. There would be little real humility. But Warren is a guy who will go out and run three miles on Sunday at midnight because he's just realized that his training log had been miscalculated. Not one to make a lot of plans, if he had one, it would be non-negotiable. Warren's stories are too quirky to be fictional. You just can't make that shit up.

My training partners and I used to go on about finding the perfect job for the serious triathlete. "It's an airline pilot," somebody would suggest. "They only work a few days each month, can take their running shoes with them on trips, and never get charged for their bike." Somebody else might suggest a firefighter (able to train while on duty), a teacher (summer off), or a lifeguard (winters off). And all of them had to do with time off or the ability to train as if training and working were distinctly and necessarily separate. The irony that the discussion took place amongst professional triathletes was not lost on the few guys in the back who actually worked regular jobs. I don't recall if there was a consensus but many years later, I would remember that working period in Dickensian fashion as both the best and worst of times. When you wake up in the morning and ask yourself, "Should I run an easy eight miles on the trails before breakfast, or should I ride up the coast with my pals and stop for lunch?"

That is revisionist thinking, of course; that decade of sore legs and unstable pay checks lost to the brighter periods and awards dinners and people knowing your name. I was more lucky than good. Still, how many times have you heard of the top age group athlete who quits a good job and has a go at The Dream only to end up over-trained, injured, unemployed, and wondering what was so terribly wrong with a good job?

Maybe their timing was wrong. Maybe they were lucky to have been smart enough or wistful enough to just go for it.

Sometimes it works that way. You got to take your shot and hope you hit something. Deal with life in the morning.

The American poet and novelist, Charles Bukowski, once created a character, *Henry Chinaski*, who suggested that "endurance is more important than truth." Never mind that Bukowski's hard charging protagonist from the short story, *Barfly*, was taking about what it takes to become a really good drunk. The lesson imbued is that if you want truth, you have to endure something to find it. You have to *work* for it. I believed Bukowski's *Chinaski* (and his other shenanigans) for a very long time, "Yep, just stick it out, man, hang in there and one day enlightenment will envelop you like morning rays through an unencumbered window."

But when I reread the short story some years later, I realized that Henry had been deluded partially by drink but mostly by a society that can't seem to wrap its head around the idea that work can be a hell of a lot of fun. Henry's truth was always there. And he had been working and drinking too hard to see it.

185

I'm not so sure that my gig as a pro triathlete ever taught me the meaning of life. I saw some meanness in competition but got to hang out with some beautiful people for a lot longer than I deserved. Maybe that's as good as it gets. Which, if you appreciate it, ain't too bad at all. It's good work, as they say, if you can get it.

====

The idea of corporate fitness took hold about the same time as the early triathlon. The early 80s brought bike racks and shower facilities to cube farms under the guise that increased worker fitness levels correlate to productivity, fewer sick days, and the success of the softball team. Hundreds of studies supported this claim. But still, there was this ideological chasm between work and play. Endurance athletes could ride their bikes to work or run at lunch and grab a quick shower but somehow you ended up paying for your play with longer hours and contemptuous glances. Perhaps the politics of guilt was more in play than any dogmatic influence from the bosses. While the fitness revolution altered the way we incorporated health into our lives, it didn't foundationally change them.

A lot of people still hate their jobs and only work out to look good in a tank top.

It took the 20-something whiz kids of the Dotcom Era to show us how work and play can and should be interfaced. Board meetings held around the ping pong table, not-when-the-surf's-up scheduling, and t-shirt dress codes hid the fact that a lot of really smart people worked some really long hours. But something happened on the way to the skate park and some cool kids discovered that at some point, you just have to show some profit to justify the party. That buzzkill messed with a lot of heads. "We were on to something," they claimed, "just needed a little bit more time ... and a new infusion of cash." Sorry, the Suits said, ping pong table is repossessed. But a new idea had been planted, a paradigm shift of pain and pleasure.

And now, in a post-millennium, recessionary period, we remain confused but hopeful about how to define and differentiate between our five to nine bike rides and our nine to five jobs. A post-COVID environment has shown us the increasingly blurred lines between work and play, between leisure and effort. Some people can't wait to retire, and others push on until they are stage-hooked off to "make room for new ideas."

Through it all, any occupational shift, particularly retirement, presents us with new kinds of rehabilitation, now opportunities for stimulation and boredom, quest and rest. So many of us are over-identified in our jobs. And then (we) go away. We miss stability, even if we hate the job.

Tom Warren, for his part, knows about missing things. In 2009, he lost his only wife to a horrible cycling accident. In 2003, he lost his self-built dream house to a raging wildfire. Through it all he kept moving, kept working at "projects" as his put it, "The things that I wake up and just start doing before I really know why." It wasn't just working or playing. He was building what some other forces had torn down; moving perpetually as a sea creature that drowns when they stop processing oxygenated water.

Warren is a craftsman in the style of a pre-Industrial Revolution MacGyver. He does his own taxes and changes his own flats. His endeavors run together as do his thoughts. He doesn't read Marx but there is no division of labor in his personal society.

Tom Warren has rebuilt the house and patched the hole in his heart. He is not an unhappy or unsatisfied man. He keeps his overhead low and his handful of ancient investments fresh. For Warren, a man who will ride his bike to Canada and back on a day's notice, there was always a kind of cold fluidity to his choices— some calculation, some risk, some thought, some thoughtlessness. Warren, the accountant with a private university pedigree, never ran the numbers too close, never thought he deserved this because he gave that. But neither was he reckless with his time and his passing tides. Therein may lie the secret to both his perspective and his perseverance. Tom Warren knew how to triage his emotions.

If Tom was going to own a dive bar, it was going to be the best crummy saloon in the city. If he was going to try endurance sports, then he might as well tackle the Ironman. And if he was going to live in the world he might as well live all the way in, blurring the lines as they challenged him. When he enters races these days, they serve as barometers, an outward judge of an inner state. There is no finish line, just boxes to check.

I have been lucky to have found gainful employment in my life after competitive sport, a job that is like rain—heavy in sound but soft to the touch. My students rarely know of my other careers, they just see a guy lecturing about sport in a way that might confuse or on occasion might thrill them. The hardest part of my job is engineering my words so that there are more of the later and less of the former. I see Tom on occasion, usually riding his bike up the coast, head bent, and eyes fixed on the distance. I don't think of him as being retired from a career because I'm not sure I could say that in any traditional sense of the word, he never had one. His balance sheet might excite a few entrepreneurs, but it is doubtful he would do anything different if shown his life in arrears on Excel.

Perhaps the measure of our work or our play is incalculable while we are engaged in either. When it's all done, someone else will come along and judge the noisy aspirations which defined us. Which is all the more reason to knock off early. Have a drink. Go for a run. Burn your computer. Turn off your bra. I know it's a cliché, but I like the imagery.

"Have you ever seen a hearse pulling a U-Haul trailer?"

Prescript: I've come to realize that if we situate ourselves too firmly in an idea, a cause, a place or a time, we will fail to grow. The period of my youth, the 60s and 70s, held its own power over me if not society in general. But it is fair to argue that any period can and will have an effect of a person's psyche. In March of 2004, I traveled to UC Berkeley to speak at a friend's funeral. But in many ways, I was finally beginning to bury parts of the rebel in my past. The trip was cathartic in many ways; a kind of slow dance in rehab by letting my youth go away. I'd been enamored with the social movements of the 60s, reveling in the ideas of freedom and justice and a dying off-of the traditions born in post-war America. But then the tumult of 1968 tossed the summer of love in the gutter. The Tet Offensive in Vietnam, campus protests, challenges with North Korea, the assassinations of MLK and RFK, the 1969 Santa Barbara oil spill, and a general global upheaval in most societies helped change my tune. But even as a pre-pubescent teen, I was glad to have felt the magnetic pull of a group/movement that thought and perhaps did for a period, change the whole fucking world. And for those wounded idealists who risked everything, the rehabilitation into something less than what they had hoped for must've been tough. The turbulent 60s did not happen in another dimension; everything before it led to that tumult and everything after was a result of that decade's incidents and accidents. I suppose that I was lucky to have been just a handful of years too young to jump into the fray with both feet, to march in protest, to burn my draft card, to put my body on the gears. I dabbled in drugs as a secret silent form of protest but that would be a gratuitous claim given the shitty dope we smoked and the airplane glue we sniffed once or twice until the headache was worse than the effect. Still, it seems like a major rehabilitation effort for those who lose their idealism or worse, yet have it snatched away by maturity and a mortgage. They end up functionally disenchanted, constantly sleeping with yesterday. A victim of grand theft soul. Everything here is true, if only in a post rebellious mind.

In Search of the Last Hippy, Approximately

> *"If you want to live outside the law you have to be honest."*
>
> —Bob Dylan

SCOTT TINLEY

Everything in here, but the sum of its parts, is real. Some of it even approaches the truth of my tongue. I was going to the funeral for a friend. But I went hunting as well.

I was going in search of the last hippy, clinging to a long patient ideal, a vibrating notion that sent me in search of hair. I wouldn't call it a mid-life crisis exactly, but my pre-Aquarius dating was haunting me. I needed to find a flower child, receive the holy sacrament of hash, if not the free love of copulatory communion. I needed to find the last hippy, approximately.

Tin Soldiers and Nixon had come and gone only to be replaced by the Executive Branch of United Chevron Nations. Pharmaceutical agents, yoga, tofu and tarot cards had all failed me. I had to go back to the few things I remembered in the mirror—May of '68 and an incense burning, pubescent punk with an older sister.

I had gone back because when I was about to be called up, I went completely sideways.

I traveled north to U.C. Berkley where there had been reports of sightings, Bigfoot in beads, day-glow posters on creosote poles, acoustic guitars slung low and slouching toward the Bethlehem of free speech. And that sweet smoke wafting west to where the sun fought the horizon.

At the "Bezerkely Information Center, a ghost-colored student with thick-bottled lenses rose from a thicker bio-text and studied me with nasally disdain.

"Hippies? Try the Discovery Channel or get-a-life.com."

There had to be one Leftist still breathing in this former bastion of political activism; just one young American who'd stand up, or sit down for what's right, or at least one '63 VW Bus driving further, further into the past. I prayed for the simple possibility.

Wandering the vast rolling beauty of the campus in search of anyone not welded to a Walkman or cellular device, the students looked so young, so studious, so ... entrepreneurial. The old stone buildings had alumni donor names freshly carved into the ancient stone façade. A small, study groups of aloof Asian kids spoke quietly among themselves. It was that sing-song diction of cyber-speak, the language of six figure starting salaries. The scattered art on the grounds that I remembered as "engaging" now looked rusted and industrial-safe. And among the spring-green redwoods, now tired and thick, their weighted branches held aloft with guywires and keep-off signs, stood newer concrete structures, re-bar gray and Molotov-proof. Where were the red slashes and yellow bandanas?

I followed the smell of fresh beans past the Hearst Library and the Zellerbach Business School towards a clean well-lighted place with the words *Free Speech Café* routed into a piece of thinly varnished plywood. The walls were papered in black and white murals of bright faces; Mario Savio with a bull horn looking angry, concerned, speaking freely. Savio had died in'96 from heart troubles. He was fifty-three, dead before he got old, electrically charged before his own somatic institution shut him down.

I read the caption and closed my eyes to hear the words:

"There is a time when the operation of the machine becomes so odious, makes you so sick at heart, that you can't take part; you can't even passively take part, and you've got to put your bodies upon the gears and upon the wheels, upon the levers, upon all the apparatus, and you've got to make it stop."

The only wheels and gears I'd put my body on when Savio delivered those words in '64 was attached to the chain on my little bicycle. The machines had changed but people were still chained to them, not knowing what for.

I took my five-dollar coffee and tried to drag a patio chair into the sun, but it was bolted to the concrete floor, and I swore under my breath. What was I here for? Oh, that's right, another eulogy, another death at 51, another good heart gone bad. It was my turn to speak in front of the Berkeley Brass about an injustice, albeit a singular one. My young friend with an old heart, Brian Maxwell, was dead. Brian had run 2:14 for the marathon, had been on the Canadian Olympic Team. Nothing wrong with his ticker.

Wrong.

He'd left a wife and six young kids in his wake, wondering. The good, they die young.

I had expected to find inspiration in the past, but all that came to me was a point of intersection where memory played leapfrog between then and now and the present became its own dimension. It was the tyranny of the urgent. Instead, I felt sick. Was there no one left who would rage against the death and dying of the tie-dyed ethos? Was it all a diethylamide dream woken by Narcan and dwindling numbers; that eve of destruction gone quietly into the dying light? Who killed Davey Jones and my friend Brian Maxwell? What hammer stopped his young and wild heart?

I marched down Telegraph Ave. past Rasputin's Records where you could once buy rolling papers that sold for a nickel, past Shakespeare and Co. where you could get a copy of *On the Road* for a buck, past the Nuevo-vendors hawking bangles that dangled and piercings in body parts I never knew were strong enough. And then up to People's Park where I imagined a crowd had taken in with me a dozen strong. But then only to realize after arriving that they'd all lit out for the bin of free clothes and pawed through the big plywood box for anything they could take and sell.

Somehow, I sensed that I might be closer. Something in the depravity gassed my cynicism and I knew the last hippy, approximately, would be here.

I scanned the bulletin board and saw an ad to make $15 an hour from your home, no plasma required. I watched a couple kiss and heard one of them complain about his lover's scratchy beard. I saw a basketball game of smack-talk and chain nets below the bent rim, but no ball. I saw people sleeping in red sawdust, spooning their lives in needles of pine and steel. I saw prom queens lost to hard times and soup lines and the bitterness of faded rouge. I saw shoeless, fatherless, fearless children on soundless swings, the bearings long since gone, and the polished metal bushings smooth and efficient.

I felt the future, but it came up cold and hard-edged against the hope of what had passed.

But there, off in the mimsy borogoves of a few pale maples stood a middle-aged man with a garden hose, real water flowing onto a young garden. He wore the tapestry of kings, a proud bed-sheet robe. And he spoke freely, concern in his intentioned eyes, his lips offering some inane immutable truth to no one save the white rabbit in his mind.

I approached him from behind and asked if he was the last, approximately. He turned slowly, not noticing that he had watered the ground below my feet.

"Tell Jann he promised me the cover," He said, "we had a deal." And then he moved back inside his garden and his pulpit.

To think about resistance is to think about acceptance. To think about rebellion is to seek rehabilitation. Not for sale or selling out. Everything is true and nothing is true. And quantum physics never did get you that four-bedroom, three bath in the burbs. War is hell but heaven has left earth, left the building with Elvis. What we have now is an iPod zeitgeist, Rollerball come true, Vacuum Ville. Everything is gone but the uncertainty of some goodness. Free love replaced with free downloads, nothing but rising temps and falling forests, endangered species replaced by pocket-pets. I don't want to live in an air-conditioned world, and I'll never learn to speak Mandarin. I'd gone to a friend's funeral, but a lot more had passed.

And these kids, the students of Cal, don't they care? Okay, previous generations didn't leave things in such great shape. But whoever really cleans a hotel room? I ain't buying that "I'm only a dot in a dot.com world" shit. It's just work, baby … just connecting the political with the personal, as someone said.

Walking back up the avenue, I was compelled to revolt at the repulsion, disgusted that I was still unable to distinguish the peace agents from the sales agent, unable to speak out against the slick genocide with a Jeffersonian air and plain old Grace. The best I could do was to jaywalk into Starbucks and take a piss without buying anything at all.

I miss the obvious ambiguity of war.

Someday I'll go there on vacation for the first time.

Yeah, me and the ghost of Hanoi Jane. Stepping over the land minds of our past. But at least I had come to be an uneasy rider over my failed ideological past. It's a start.

Prescript: The short piece below was catalyzed by yet another boring New Year's Eve. There was the usual festive spirit but there seemed a low-lying malaise in the air that was equal parts, regret, hope, and nostalgia. The COVID crisis had passed, the economy was strong, we were out of Afghanistan ... but still. When I finished the piece, I realized nothing had been said. And when I went to hit "delete," I realized that was my point exactly. The passing of time is likely the only egalitarian kind of loss—it happens to everyone regardless of their age, sex, religion, class, ethnicity or country of origin. And when it's gone, it ain't coming back regardless of your yoga class or anti-aging creams. I envy people who seem to be just fine, thank you, as they age up and their skin falls, as their intellect shrinks and their waistlines grow, gracefully surrendering those things of youth. And those who keep talking about living in the moment while talking about their next job promotion? Or worse yet, the ones who tell you to constantly stay in the here and now as they take cell phone calls from anywhere but where they are? Conflicted bastards. The smarter ones realize the troubling ambiguity of New Year's and get married on January 1st or figure out how to have their birthdays on the first day of the year. It gives them a reason to celebrate or at least take their mind off the fact that they are one year closer to the end than the beginning. I am vowing to make this next New Year's Eve better than before. I'm not sure how; maybe I'll just skip the whole day and start next year on January 2nd. At least I have some time to think about it.

Where the Echoes Keep Calling

I've been thinking about the things I missed these past few years. Maybe it's a sign of age. Or maybe it's been the dreary weather or the passing of my rock and roll heroes. Perhaps it was just something I ate. My mother missed things. The old and the criminally nostalgic miss things. But I don't want to miss things because I don't want to be nostalgic, and I don't want to be old.

Generally, I'd rather live in the present. But I am getting older, regardless of my ability to lie about my age. And I need—not want—to remember.

As another year goes under the bridge, we are reminded of significant decades past; first in 10s, then 20s, and suddenly it's been 40 years and we are hopeless to reflect on those times and places and people who informed and shaped our youth. And we miss those times not for the sense that time is running away on us, but for the loss of everything those delicious years gave us.

We triage out the crap. Happily forgetting the struggles and the pain and dead batteries and the death of a good dog and your roommate drank your last beer. Quite selectively—and in service of our health and happiness—we negotiate what we remember and what we miss.

As athletes, we miss how we held our young bodies up against an older world. How we could recover from a workout with a 30-minute nap. How we could handle second helpings. How we could justify a bike that costs more than a car. How we were immortal.

I sometimes wonder how the artist or the academic or the mercantilist or the mother or the soldier holds themselves up against the ravages of time and tide. Does a painter miss an original they sold to pay the rent? Does a scientist miss that discovery born on youthful energy and countless lab hours? Does the trader miss the jouissance of the deal that brought them wealth if not happiness? The mother sending her youngest off the college; the soldier in peacetime; the retiring athlete, the rebel with no cause?

=====

The last decade was rife with years of transition, of conflict, of change. As the COVID crisis eased, tensions between the U.S. and China increased. The effects of climate change were becoming increasingly evident. Peace in Ethiopia, war in Ukraine. Geopolitical shifts toward human rights, the return of inflation. Argentina's World Cup victory helping to unify Latin America, turmoil in British politics. One could argue David Byrne's "same as it ever was" or Ecclesiastes' "a time for every purpose under heaven." But neither pop culture nor biblical references can explain the permanence of change.

Still, shit happens. And the past few years were no exception. So, we are beholden to remember because that act informs, educates, and offers a chance to do better. Or at least a chance to try.

There is a built-in hopefulness of a new year. Nobody wishes for a fucked-up future. There is work to be done, though. Plenty of it. As Eliot reminds us in The Hollow Men, "Between the idea and the reality falls the shadow." Here's to running towards the light, of doing the work, of remembering the good, the bad, and the ugly and dealing with each in way that moves us in a positive direction.

Another trip around the sun and the people who we want on our train.

Prescript: When I left a fifteen-year career as a professional athlete, I struggled to find a suitable new occupation. Nothing got me up early. After a few false starts and plenty of vacuous nights, I went back to grad school and started working on the beach as a lifeguard again—good gigs but perhaps not for a forty-year-old with kids and a mortgage. The essay below reflects on how a decline in one's sporting abilities, if not loss of a physical life, comes fraught with its own challenges. I suppose the power of sport is immutable. But so is anything we do that requires an all-or-nothing approach. It seems that many people struggle with a loss of or change in career. When I retired from sport, I had a very difficult year, wondering "what's next?" "What is the next chapter, and can I be the author of that text?" I saw too many of my fellow retired athletes struggle with issues of self-worth, finances, health, direction, friendship, and identity. I loved and appreciated my family, but I felt that I was born with a warrior's heart—the need to be needed. The idea of a beleaguered domesticity scared me into an early grave. My answer was to study the transition, the rehabilitation back into a degree of happiness if not basic satisfaction. Along the way I found that the two significant analogues for life transition were the empty-nested mother (whose identity was rolled up into raising her children) and the soldier returning from theaters of war (I was dodging bullets, fearing for my life but at least I felt more alive than sitting on my parents couch in Nebraska with a quart of Jack Daniels watching re-runs of Happy Days). This is but one of my attempts to make sense of this largely under-appreciated issue that nearly everyone faces at some point in their life. It might be graduation from high school, it might be breaking up with a significant other, and it might be growing old and fat and lazy. No one is immune from life's nuanced challenges and opportunities to return better, stronger, smarter. And more accepting of themselves and the new world around them.

A Sport to Steer By

I've told this story before. I wove it as a personal embellishment, something to fit the mold of my mood at that time. It wasn't a lie then. But now, when I feel my tongue up against the truth, I know it's better the second time around. It stretches out beyond the light and shade of fiction. Right into life, right into sport. Better, like leftovers. Marinated fact.

We had stepped outside into the clear night, leaving behind the sterile bank of fluorescent light and the cyber-smell of Pentium processors. Several students lit cigarettes, chatted in muted tones trying to sound worldly. It was the fall of 1999, less than ninety days before the new millennium when the world was supposed to end and Jesus would return, ivory white iPod earbuds dangling below his golden crown. "There wasn't much time," everyone said. Store up water and batteries and ammo and pray like the winged-one.

Of course, all that ensued was a 200-point gain on the Dow.

What did I care, though? I was trying to reinvent myself, regardless of if there would be a world to inhabit.

Our professor had said *"ten minute break only, please, there's much to do."* Fair enough, I thought, wooden desks were a lot more comfortable than a weight-saving carbon fiber seat post and five-hour bike rides had oddly trained me well for three-hour classes. I was back in grad school because that's where I had left off, I told myself, before going off to sport as if I had gone off to war. There were similarities. More than I knew. And if the Second Coming was going to happen, as a writer and a believer, I was sure that the Man wouldn't use this cliché'd date to download his return.

Some guy, dressed mostly in black, his sideburns straining for youthful style, working overtime toward coolness, tapped his cigarettes deftly so that only one would protrude, phallically, and pushed it in my direction. I must've looked at him oddly, like people stare at a pimple and will themselves to move their eyes away.

What's wrong, this kid asked me, don't smoke this brand?

No, that's not it at all. I watched my foot tap and fell into the poignancy of the moment. It's just that I don't think anyone has ever offered me a cigarette before. He must've thought I was lying but I'd never been speaking the truth more clearly. It wasn't my fault that the kid couldn't see I was quietly; desperately trying to connect the life of an athlete to, well, to everyone else. In hindsight, I wish I would've taken the protruding tobacco even if to put it behind my ear, James Dean with an airbag, so that I could validate my act of remembrance and admit that I'd been welcomed into the diasporic netherworld.

It was an innocent and benevolent gesture by someone younger than me, someone trying to get old quickly because a certain *hardening* was en vogue. He had no idea of my background in sport. I had no idea of his in, well, whatever it was that formed him in the time before then. He could've been a great jockey or a ranked boxer, a dancer or a poet.

The anonymity felt liberating, felt like the world didn't need to be framed around end zones and baselines and it was okay because life had its own start and finish lines. I used to think that sport existed as one great metaphor for everything else, that life could be studied by living a sporting existence, a pen and paper in my back pocket. And then for a while, I thought I might've had it backwards, the sport and life part. Maybe things like education and work and relationships were more than allegorical preparation for a world that began with a playground ball, a pair of running shoes and a coach saying, "C'mon out here and play, kid."

In hindsight, I realized that the lines became blurred because I allowed them to, even willing them to fuzz in some self-serving vehicle of personal justification for the time and effort and ultimate identification of all that sport had been to me. I wasn't playing some game of swim, bike, and run; wasn't a soft child stuck in a man's hardening body—my sport was my life, they didn't happen in different dimensions, there was no schizophrenia, no fifty yard split of ethos and ethic. I hadn't been to the Crossroads to deal for my skill and fortune; I was doing what came naturally to live a physical life.

I was happy.

But now, regardless of what I study or teach my own students, I embrace that truer truth on the cusp where sport and life are a kind of reciprocal, a semiotic and symbiotic bathroom mirror. And when you go beyond what cultural clarity resides in the language, they don't share anything huge and permanent and fixed, they are just subsets of each other—sport is the kind of life that people choose, and life is a kind of game that people play.

The action-hero philosophers will tell us that life is about experiences, feelings, successes, and failures. It is the sum of smoke and deception, purpose and direction, love and hate, yin-yang and you fill in the gaps. Being born is a cool thing but we can't make the dead become undead. For the layperson on that arcing continuum, a trophy would be nice, something simple and validating, something to show their grandkids.

These are not unattainable concepts for people who are drawn to a raw and pure form of sport rather than the other mine fields of life; that Halliburton zeitgeist, the new tyranny of the datasphere. But you could also live a sedate and vicarious existence and if it's your truth and you're happy, who can argue? You don't need a championship ring to live fulfilled. A pop-top from an old cola will do if it has significance.

In our naivete of youth, our halcyon days before the weight of age tries to pull down our dreams with our waistlines, we circle the track and feel the soft rubber under our feet and smell the fresh cut grass as we temporarily enslave ourselves to the stopwatch. Each lap has meaning, we tell ourselves, each lap is quicker, deeper into our goal. But what do we really know at 14, or 18 or 24? What have we been conditioned to believe? Is it something tangible, alluring, 30 days the same as cash, operators are standing by? Or something still fresh and unnameable? Something cerebral or somatic that requires an investment?

In my own freshman fame, in that time when I wanted things I would never get and got things that I never wanted, I must've known that I was both a passenger and pilot, that while I was building a body and building a life, there were things beyond my control—my life flying IFR.

As athletes we develop these skills, these tendencies to draw up psychological barriers that rise beyond the biological. And even if they are smoke signals harboring things to come, we don't read them, just go around the track one more time, harder now because the guru-jock-of-the-month with a new book says that fitness is more than health, and if we must have an addiction, than what better habit to be enslaved to? This sporting life, we are convinced, is the only life.

I remember the exact moment when I had crossed the line between training for performance' sake and training for training's sake, when sport had become my life but also a kind of slow dance with death at the same time. Oh, there was balance, but it came as two junk yard dogs circling each other.

It was during the birth of our first child, my wife in the jaws of a protracted but not entirely uncomfortable labor. I pulled the doc aside and asked him if I had time to sneak outside for a quick five-miler. I would stay on the hospital grounds. I promised. That memory haunts me still, how I had folded myself tightly into sport and that part so far away from life itself that the only satisfaction is the audience of one and the cackling laughter you hear in the background can only be the devil.

No athlete can hide forever behind the thinly veiled excuse of ignorance. No different than anyone can hide from burnout, fatigue, malaise, and the cold harsh reality that one gig is over. Time to move on.

At least we should know when too much is too much, or too little is not enough. Still, if we see sport and life as one, it is a great task to distinguish the map from the territory, to differentiate a training program from a training lifestyle, to know a chance to determine if we can still hit the outside jump shot, that Vahalik playground where we meet up with some old buddies. And for the moment, the clock has stopped.

Sport is a drug. But so is life. The needle slips when you slip out of your mother's womb. There is a terrifying excitement where part of you wants to go back into the shade and the other wants to jump into the light. You tell yourself that you just don't know, man. How could you? So, you follow your instinct to move because somehow, it's born with you, this knowledge that something possessed never has the same value or pull as it does in pursuit.

We're all hooked to some degree. It's certainly not hard to extol the virtue of sport. Simple, really. Bang away at the keys, chat up a stranger on a plane or convince a relative over for Christmas dinner that sport is good, that it's different; it allows us a chance to stand out.

From where, they ask.

From here, silly. Anywhere but right here, doing nothing.

With your sport, you tell them, you can glow in the dark. And you'd be right.

That's the bad part of the drug—it can bend a reality, squiggly lines on a desert horizon. Mirage goes from noun to verb. You glow when you're supposed to fade.

201

But statistics are our ammo, and the media is our ally. Numbers never lie and neither do heroes. It's all so believable because we want to believe it. Sportsmanship, camaraderie, physical health, goal attainment, self-knowledge—they're all there inside of sport, neatly packaged sometimes, raw and unwieldy at others. Sport provides a constellation of possibilities, and we could be a star in our own galaxy. Oh God, it's so easy—twinkle, twinkle and I won my age group and another twinkle and if only I didn't have this job I could've made The Show, could've stepped right into that aristocracy of fa**me:** a fat house, a skinny wife, the UPS driver calling me by my first name.

Go for it, *IT* says, grab the brass ring and find yourself separated from life and don't worry about separating from yourself. When you return, you're just a post-traumatic game show away from the normalcy of a remote control and sixer of plain wrap.

Athletes and athletics have become a fixture in our culture, socializing our youth, teaching them valuable lessons not so easily taught at home or in the classroom. They also clog up Sunday afternoons when the commentary clones are clogging our minds with flashy media dribble poured out *up close and personal.* As fan-addicts, sport thrills us like few institutions can, often over-shadowing theater, the arts, music and war-for-profit as the chosen form of entertainment. Not since the Roman Empire has sport played such a role in how we live our lives. Is it because commercial sport remains the last form in which the ending is still a mystery?

What role and what mystery though? Chomsky has said that sport keeps people from worrying about things that matter to their lives. Indeed, we are acculturated through sport in ways we must be wary of; dominate powers slipping bourgeoisie ideology into Super Bowl half time shows. And not a journalist in the house willing to point out that Janet's exposed breast was itself manufactured.

=====

I may have begun this song as the naïve troubadour many years ago but now, even after the wounds of re-entry have healed, I wonder if I had subversively and in sequence convinced myself that it is the game that gives us life? That play comes before players, events before eventuality and sport before spirit. Yes, there is no situational ethos riding shotgun in arrear when I say that my life of sport has become bigger than a life of life.

The Native American belief that dreams are wiser than men, it can't be denied. Though I never dreamed of becoming a champion, of winning races around the world, traveling on the corporate meal ticket of sponsors, I sometimes lie awake deciphering the chasm code between a grainy, idealized recollection of sport's virtues and the dreams I had of being happily married with happy kids and happy dinners together.

Balancing meant the ability to hold my line around a tight corner at 30 mph. Fulfillment referred to race results and frequent flyer miles. But I cannot take back what I gave any more than I can return what was given me. And I cannot put sunscreen on retroactively. Sport was life at the time, which made it true, if only for that time. To deny the Campbellian call would've put me in a zero-sum suburb, breathing shallow stucco, drinking month-old chardonnay from a box. The same could be said for a divorce or a joining AA when you are finally ready.

I suppose that it's like the pitcher who's ahead by one run in the seventh inning and the crowd, the manager, hell everybody still thinks he still has the stuff to bring it. And then he takes himself out of the game; just doesn't show up at the top of the eighth. Nobody can really know what he's thinking or why he handed the ball over. But you have to know that he's looking at the game, *his* game, from a new perspective, a place that has its own form of irony attached. A place you can't really describe to someone who hasn't earned it but loves and hates you more than you will know in that moment.

My mistake was that I took myself out of the game after it was over and the stadium was dark and quiet. Sometimes though, you do your best thinking in the dark, with ghosts guiding your thoughts.

But sport and our exit from it must be studied beyond the convenience of mutual détente where one is big and the other small and you have to hold them up to a mirror to figure out which is which. Any formal discourse would include an analysis of its conflict as well as its charisma.

Either way, sport can become a way of looking at life, a way both to filter and objectify your own experience; a reference point by which to judge your headway or rate of decline, a lifeline to hold on to as the earth swallows everything else around you or a golden calf that you chase into the promise of the abyss. Joe-bag-of-donuts or Joe DiMaggio, sport is your lighthouse or your barrier reef.

Until it's not.

Long before advanced global positioning systems allowed satellites to tell us where we are, there was a simple form of seaman's navigation called deduced reckoning. It required a chart of the local waters, a reliable compass, and an accurate timepiece. All that you needed to know was where you'd started, what your direction of travel was and how long it was taking you as you plotted your position on a line drawn on the chart. Simple stuff, unless you changed direction or speed and then you started a new line from a new point on the chart. If you became distracted by a pretty sunset, a prettier face or a frosty boat drink, you had to go below decks and start a new line every time. It's tedious, not entirely accurate, and reliant on things that are easily confused; things like where did you *really* start and what time *is* it, anyway?

The average person will create these markers on the yardstick of their existence out of significant events; life-changing occurrences like births and new jobs and graduations and weddings and then deaths. Every section of the greeting card rack is covered. But if you look beyond the event itself then you will notice that it attains its import due to the significance of someone entering or exiting your life.

But that happens all the time; you don't need a 40th birthday party to feel the pleasure or the pain, the love or the loss of connection to others.

The same is true for sport. Yeah, it's more than a game, maybe a passion or a career ... it's a heavily peopled marker.

As athletes we have the advantage of looking at sport as a continuous series of markers that include the people on our journey who bore witness to major events. Take away the people and the events still exist, but not really. These social constructs serve as cornerstones: our first soccer goal, making the high school track team, a 10k personal record, the first and the most recent of everything physical. Nobody wants to think about the end of anything. Athletes like to think only of going forward, sometimes sideways but never back and never, ever stop. Because forward means more people, deeper relationships, better understanding. We must know that, even if we don't know it.

Rehab into a new occupation takes resiliency. Letting go takes work.

And I suppose that each time we pause, not stopping but slowing down enough to take new bearings, we must also ponder our direction, our means and our purpose. The decisions from there are based on what we know about our place in sport and our place in life. And the people who make the events valid. They flow together like water, one no different from the other.

I should've taken the cigarette and put it in my pocket. I should've put out my hand, said "Thanks but I don't smoke." I should've asked him if he was a painter and where

he'd had his nose pierced. I just didn't know.

EPILOGUE

This collection was intended to remind us that to restore is to commit to a hardscrabble apprenticeship. A sometime whirlwind transition with hopeful outcomes and no guarantees; a timeless period in one's life when we have choices but are not in control. When we exist in a temporary state of movement that pings and caroms but rarely goes tilt.

As has been suggested, rehabilitation is about getting better. Sometimes more, sometimes less.

I felt both blessed and cursed to form this text while my own heart was reforming itself. I hope this collection shines some light on the many and varied issues faced when life goes south, when we ask that perennial question, "Why me?" I hope you find something relevant, close to home, even if it conjures uneasy feelings. I hope these stories, essays, and interviews reminded you that you are not alone in your struggles. And I hope you find empathy for yourself and others as they climb back towards the light.

I know it sounds awkward, but I wish no one felt compelled to read this book. Perhaps that might signal that the non-reader had never fully encountered nor felt faced with the vagaries of rehabilitation in its many and varied forms. But life just ain't like that for most of us. And so, we endeavor to improve our lot in life with the help of family, friends, science, patience, work, education, spirituality, sex, drugs, rock and roll, and plain old dumb luck.

... and to be a better soul on the other side of rehab.

—S.T.

www.ingramcontent.com/pod-product-compliance
Lightning Source LLC
Chambersburg PA
CBHW071546200326
41519CB00021BB/6633